Dementia Caregiver's Guide

Help Without Guesswork: Practical Support for Dementia—No Doctor Talk, No False Promises

Natalie Mills

Copyright

Cover Design by Natalie Mills

ISBN (Paperback): 978-1-923524-18-7
ISBN (Hardcover): 978-1-923524-19-4

Epigraph

The Doorway

Sometimes you are not the one who stays.
You are the one who arrives,
holding the space for a little while.

An hour.
An afternoon.
A weekend.

May this book help those who step through that doorway -
offering practical care, steady presence,
and help without guesswork.

Dedication

Two Sisters, One Truth

For my Auntie Phyllis and my Nanny,
two sisters who walked two very different paths through Dementia
and unknowingly taught me the same truth.

Nothing was ever wrong with you.
What was missing was confidence, calm, and courage in the people who loved you.

This book is written in your honour -
and for every family still learning
that fear does far more harm than memory loss ever could.

Contents

Introduction

You Don't Need to Be Perfect to Help

If you've picked up this book, chances are someone you care about is living with dementia, and you want to help - but you're not quite sure how.

Maybe you're the adult child who lives several hours away and visits on weekends. Maybe you're the neighbor who's noticed your dear friend struggling and wants to offer an afternoon of support. Maybe you're part of a local church community where someone needs a few hours of companionship each week. Or maybe you're the family member who gets called when the primary caregiver needs to run errands, attend appointments, or simply take a well-earned break.

If any of this sounds familiar, you're probably feeling something else too: a mixture of willingness and worry that you will get it wrong. You want to step in. You want to be useful. But there's that nagging voice asking, "What if I do something wrong? What if I make things worse? What if I don't know what to do when something goes sideways?"

Here's what I want you to understand right from the start: that worry doesn't disqualify you from helping. In fact, it tells us something important about you: you care enough to want to get it right.

But here's the thing about helping someone with dementia that might surprise you: getting it "right" has very little to do with having all the answers, and everything to do with showing up with calm presence and genuine care.

This book isn't about turning you into a professional caregiver. It's not about teaching you to manage complex medical situations or navigate the long-term journey of dementia care. This book is about something much simpler and, in many ways, much more valuable: helping you step in confidently for short periods - an hour, an afternoon, a weekend - without the fear that holds so many willing helpers back.

Why This Book Exists

The inspiration for this book came from witnessing the same scene play out countless times: caring people who genuinely want to help, but who hold back because they're afraid of doing the wrong thing. I've seen adult children hesitate to visit their parents because they don't know how to handle repetitive questions. I've watched neighbors tentatively offer help, then retreat when they encounter confusion or agitation. I've spoken with church members who want to provide respite for overwhelmed caregivers but worry they're not qualified.

The truth is, most of the time, the fear is bigger than the actual challenge.

What people living with dementia need most from their helpers isn't medical expertise or perfect responses to every situation. What they need is someone who can remain calm when things feel uncertain, offer gentle presence when confusion arises, and maintain dignity and kindness even when communication becomes difficult.

These aren't professional skills. These are human skills.

And if you're someone who cares enough to worry about doing right by a person with dementia, you likely already have more of these skills than you realize.

This book exists to bridge the gap between wanting to help and feeling confident enough to actually do it. It's designed to take the mystery out of short-term dementia support and replace anxiety with practical, gentle guidance that works in real-world situations.

Who This Book Is For

This book is written specifically for what I call "stepping-in helpers" - people who want to provide meaningful support for someone with dementia during short visits or care periods.

You might be:

- An adult child who visits regularly but feels uncertain during those visits
- A family member who gets called to help when the primary caregiver needs a break
- A friend or neighbor who wants to offer practical support but doesn't know where to start

- A church or community member looking to provide respite care
- Someone who cares deeply but has limited experience with dementia
- A person who wants to help but worries about making mistakes or causing distress

This book is perfect for you if:

- You want to help for specific periods rather than provide ongoing daily care
- You're looking for practical, simple guidance that doesn't require medical training
- You want to feel confident stepping in without fear of doing the wrong thing
- You need reassurance that your help matters, even if it feels small

What Makes This Book Different

Most books about dementia are written either for medical professionals or for primary caregivers managing the full scope of long-term care. This book fills a different need entirely.

It's designed for short-term help. Rather than covering the entire landscape of dementia care, this book focuses specifically on what matters when you're stepping in for limited periods. You'll learn what to prioritize during a two-hour visit versus a weekend stay, and what you can safely let go of when your time is brief.

It emphasizes presence over perfection. You won't find complex care protocols or medical procedures here. Instead, you'll discover that the most meaningful help often comes from simply being calm, consistent, and kind. This book will show you how powerful your steady presence can be, even when you don't have all the answers.

It gives you permission to be imperfect. Perhaps most importantly, this book operates from the understanding that helpful doesn't mean flawless. You'll find reassurance throughout these pages that making small mistakes doesn't undo the good you're doing, and that caring intention matters more than perfect execution.

What You'll Learn

This book will take you from uncertainty to confidence in your ability to provide meaningful short-term support. Here's what lies ahead:

Understanding what dementia actually looks like from a helper's perspective - not the clinical descriptions you might have read elsewhere, but the day-to-day realities you're likely to encounter during your visits.

Communication approaches that actually soothe rather than agitate, along with practical ways to handle repetition and confusion without losing your patience or creating stress for either of you.

Gentle assistance with personal care when it's needed, eating challenges that might arise, and how to work with routines and familiar comforts to create calm, positive experiences.

What to do when emotions rise - both theirs and yours - including guidance for those challenging moments when anxiety, agitation, or sadness surface during your time together.

Stage-specific support that acknowledges how dementia changes over time, so you'll know what matters most during early-stage visits, mid-stage periods when confusion increases, and later stages when presence becomes more important than conversation.

Throughout every chapter, you'll find real-world scenarios and gentle guidance for those moments when things don't go as planned. You'll learn when and how to step back without guilt, discover ways to support the primary caregiver beyond just helping with direct care, and understand what truly counts as helping - even when your contribution feels small.

Your Caring Heart Is Your Greatest Qualification

Before we dive into the practical guidance, I want to address the elephant in the room: the feeling that you're not qualified to help someone with dementia.

Maybe you're thinking you don't have enough experience, or you don't know enough about the condition, or you're worried you'll say the wrong thing at the wrong time. Maybe you've heard stories about dementia care that made it sound impossibly complex, or you've had a brief encounter that left you feeling out of your depth.

Here's what I've learned from a lifetime of witnessing both professional and family dementia care: the most meaningful help rarely comes from having perfect knowledge or flawless technique. It comes from showing up with genuine care and the willingness to stay calm when things feel uncertain.

The person you're helping doesn't need you to be a dementia expert. They need you to be a caring human being who can sit with them when they're confused, speak gently when they're agitated, and maintain their dignity when they're struggling. They need someone who won't rush them, won't correct every mistake, and won't treat them like they're broken.

If you care enough to have picked up this book, you already have the most important qualification: a heart that wants to help.

Everything else can be learned.

And that's exactly what this book is designed to teach you, in simple, reassuring terms that acknowledge your caring intention while building your practical confidence.

The person with dementia in your life needs helpers like you - people who care enough to show up, even when it feels uncertain. They need your willingness to be present, your gentle patience, and your commitment to treating them with dignity and kindness.

You don't need to be perfect to make a real difference in someone's life. You just need to be willing to try, armed with some practical guidance and the reassurance that your caring presence matters more than you might imagine.

So take a breath, let go of the pressure to get everything right, and let's begin this journey together. By the time you finish this book, you'll have everything you need to step in confidently, knowing that your help - imperfect as it might sometimes feel - is both valuable and deeply appreciated.

The Hour, Afternoon, Weekend Overview

If You're Helping for an Hour	If You're Helping for an Afternoon	If You're Helping for a Weekend
• Greet with warmth and patience. • Observe the current mood... • Offer a simple activity or help with a task. • Leave calmly, with reassurance.	• Spend time together, unrushed. • Share a meal or go for a walk. • Assist with routines or light chores. • Bring a bit of comfort and familiarity.	• Learn routines and care tips. • Plan calming activities. • Give breaks to the primary caregiver. • Be flexible and kind to yourself.

What Dementia Really Looks Like Day-to-Day

When Dementia Becomes Human Again

WHEN DAISY FIRST AGREED to spend Saturday afternoons with her neighbor Gregory, she had prepared herself for something dramatic. She'd read about memory loss and confusion online, imagining she'd need to constantly redirect him or manage crisis moments. Instead, she found herself sitting at his kitchen table, listening to the same story about his garden three times while they shared biscuits. It was repetitive, yes, but it wasn't frightening. It was just... ordinary.

Dementia in daily life rarely looks like the dramatic portrayals we see in films or read about in medical descriptions. It's much more subtle, much more human, and often much more manageable than people expect.

The day-to-day reality includes:

- Conversations that circle back to familiar topics rather than complete confusion

· Moments of clarity mixed with moments of uncertainty, often within the same hour

· Everyday activities that continue, just perhaps at a different pace or with small adaptations

· Preferences and personality traits that remain remarkably consistent

The reality is that people living with dementia are still themselves. They still enjoy a cup of tea, still have preferences about what to watch on television, and still respond to kindness and patience. The medical diagnosis doesn't erase the person you're helping - it just means some things work differently now.

What You'll Actually See

Morning routines might take longer, but they still happen. Gregory may forget what day it is, but he remembers how he likes his coffee. Daisy might struggle with new names, but she lights up when talking about her grandchildren from decades ago. These aren't broken people - they're people adapting to changes in how their minds process information.

Memory works in layers, and dementia affects these layers differently. Recent memories often become harder to access, while older memories can remain vivid and detailed. This means the person you're helping might not remember exactly what they had for breakfast, but they can tell you exactly how their mother made apple pie in 1952.

The confusion isn't constant. People with dementia have good days and difficult days, clear moments and foggy ones. Understanding this pattern helps you adjust your expectations and responses throughout your time together.

The Surprising Continuity

What catches many helpers off guard is how much stays the same. Personal habits, food preferences, and emotional responses often remain unchanged. Daisy still reaches for her favorite sweater. Gregory still chuckles at the same type of jokes. Their core personality shines through, even when memory falters.

Social skills often persist longer than people expect. Many individuals with dementia can carry on conversations, express opinions, and maintain relationships. They might repeat themselves or lose track of details, but the human connection remains strong and meaningful.

Moving Beyond Fear

This understanding changes everything about how you approach helping. Instead of walking into a medical situation, you're simply spending time with another person who happens to process things differently. The fear of saying the wrong thing or making mistakes begins to fade when you realize that patience and kindness matter more than perfect technique.

Your presence and genuine care make a difference in ways that extend far beyond managing symptoms. When you see dementia as part of the human experience rather than a complete transformation, you'll find yourself more relaxed and effective as a helper.

This shift in perspective sets the foundation for everything else we'll explore in this book.

Reality Check for Brief Helper Visits

Most helpers worry they'll walk into chaos or a constant crisis. The truth is far more ordinary. During a typical short visit, you're more likely to encounter someone pleased to see you, perhaps a bit uncertain about the time of day, and happy to have gentle company.

What Actually Happens During Short Visits

Your afternoon or weekend with someone living with dementia will probably include:

- Repetitive questions that aren't distressing to them, even if they feel awkward to you
- Simple activities that can be shared: folding, washing, looking through photo albums, watching familiar television programs
- Peaceful moments where very little needs to happen at all
- Conversations that drift between past and present without requiring correction

Harrison had been nervous about staying with his aunt for an entire afternoon. He'd imagined needing to constantly engage her or manage difficult behaviors. Instead, he found himself helping her sort through a box of old greeting cards - the same cards they'd sorted the week before. She was content, he was useful, and the afternoon passed quietly. Later, he realized this was exactly what help looked like: not dramatic intervention, but simple presence.

The Rhythm of Real Life

Dementia doesn't eliminate normal human rhythms. People still get tired in the afternoon, still enjoy their favorite snacks, and still have preferences about how they spend their time. Your role isn't to fix or change anything - it's to flow with these natural patterns and provide companionship along the way.

Many helpers are surprised by how much ordinary life continues. Hope spent her Saturday morning with her neighbor, expecting to manage confusion and disorientation. Instead, they made toast together, discussed the weather, and watched birds at the feeder. Her neighbor asked the same question about the birds three times, but the conversation felt natural and pleasant.

The repetition that characterizes dementia rarely feels urgent or distressing to the person experiencing it. They're not usually aware they've asked the same question multiple times. This means you can respond naturally, each time, without feeling frustrated or needing to point out the repetition.

Adjusting Your Expectations

Brief helpers often worry about filling time productively. This misses the point entirely. The goal isn't entertainment or stimulation - it's companionship and security. Sometimes the most helpful thing you can do is sit quietly together, perhaps folding towels or watching television.

Activities don't need to be complex or meaningful in traditional ways. Harrison discovered that his father-in-law enjoyed sorting coins from a jar, even though he'd forget what he was doing halfway through. The activity itself provided structure and purpose for those moments, which was enough.

The Gift of Low-Key Help

One of dementia's unexpected aspects is how it can slow life down to a gentler pace. Without the pressure to remember details or maintain complex conversations, you might find these visits surprisingly relaxing. The urgency that drives much of modern life becomes unnecessary.

This doesn't mean nothing matters or that your time lacks purpose. Rather, it means the purpose shifts from doing to being. Your calm presence provides stability and connection that extends beyond your visit hours.

Understanding this reality changes how you prepare for and approach your role as a helper. Instead of bracing for difficulty, you can look forward to a simple human connection. This shift in perspective makes you more effective and the experience more enjoyable for everyone involved.

When Reality Hits New Helpers

Even with the best intentions, certain moments can catch new helpers off guard. These aren't emergencies - they're just the small, human realities of how dementia affects daily life. Knowing what might happen helps you respond calmly rather than in panic.

Common Surprises That Catch New Helpers Off Guard

During your time helping, you might encounter:

· Clothes worn in unusual combinations or familiar routines done in a different order

· Stories shared as if they're happening now, even when they're from decades ago

· Moments when they don't recognize familiar objects or forget your name, followed by moments of perfect clarity

· Questions about people who died years ago, asked as if they might visit today

The key is understanding that these moments aren't problems you need to solve. They're simply part of how someone's brain is working today. Your job isn't to correct or fix - it's to stay calm and kind.

Isabella was startled when her father-in-law answered the door wearing his pajama top with dress trousers and formal shoes. Her first instinct was to suggest he change, but then she noticed he seemed comfortable and happy. Nothing was unsafe or undignified. She realized that sometimes, letting things be is the kindest response of all.

When Time Gets Fluid

People with dementia often experience time differently from how we do. Past events can feel immediate and present, while recent events fade quickly. Charles might tell you about his wedding day as if it happened last week, complete with vivid details and fresh emotions. This isn't confusion - it's his brain accessing memories that feel real and current to him.

Don't feel compelled to correct the timeline. If Eleanor mentions that she needs to pick up her children from school, and those children are now adults with their own families, you don't need to provide a reality check. Simply acknowledge her concern: "Tell me about your children," or "What are they like?" This validates her feelings without creating conflict.

The Doorknob Moment

Margaret experienced what many helpers encounter - the moment when someone doesn't recognize a common object. Her neighbor stared at a doorknob for several seconds, seeming genuinely puzzled about how it worked. Margaret's impulse was to explain or demonstrate. Still, instead, she gently guided her neighbor's hand and let muscle memory take over. The recognition returned naturally.

These moments can feel frightening to witness, but they're usually brief and not distressing to the person experiencing them. The brain finds alternative pathways, and familiar actions often return without intervention.

Emotional Weather Patterns

Moods can shift quickly and without obvious triggers. Robert was chatting pleasantly with his aunt when she suddenly became tearful, asking for her mother. Five minutes later, she was laughing at something on television. These emotional changes aren't your fault, and you don't need to fix them.

Think of emotions like weather patterns - they come and go naturally. Your steady presence provides the stability that helps someone weather these internal storms.

Building Confidence Through Experience

Each small surprise you handle successfully builds your confidence as a helper. You'll start recognizing patterns and developing instincts about when to respond and when to simply be present. Diana found that after several visits, she stopped worrying about saying the perfect thing and focused on maintaining a calm, accepting atmosphere.

These real-life moments teach you something crucial: helping someone with dementia is less about managing their condition and more about accepting their current experience with grace and kindness.

When Every Visit Tells a Different Story

One of the most important things to understand is that dementia isn't static. The person you're helping might be chatty and engaged during one visit, then quieter or more confused the next. This doesn't mean you did something wrong or that their condition has suddenly worsened - it just means today is different from yesterday.

The Natural Rhythm of Good Days and Hard Days

During your visits, you'll encounter:

- Energy levels and clarity that can vary significantly from day to day or even hour to hour

· External factors like weather, sleep, or minor illness that affect how someone feels and behaves

· Moments of sharp awareness followed by periods of confusion, sometimes within the same afternoon

· Your role remains the same regardless: to provide a calm, consistent presence

Understanding this variability helps you adjust your expectations and respond appropriately. On good days, you might have lovely conversations and accomplish small tasks together. On more difficult days, you might simply sit quietly and offer gentle reassurance. Both types of visits are valuable.

Marcus noticed that his grandmother was much more talkative and engaged on sunny days when she'd slept well the night before. On rainy days when she seemed tired, she preferred to sit quietly with a cup of tea, sometimes holding his hand. He learned to follow her lead rather than trying to maintain the same energy every visit. The quiet days became just as meaningful as the chatty ones.

Reading the Day's Tone

Within the first few minutes of your visit, you'll usually sense what kind of day it is. Some people wake up feeling more alert and social, while others wake up feeling foggy or withdrawn. Neither is wrong - they're just different starting points for your time together.

On engaged days, the person you're helping might remember your name immediately, ask about your family, or want to show you something important. These are wonderful opportunities for deeper connection, but don't expect every visit to follow this pattern.

When Confusion Feels Heavier

Some days, the fog of confusion seems thicker. Patricia found her neighbor staring out the window, unable to remember why she was there or what day it was. Instead of trying to orient her to reality, Patricia simply sat beside her and commented on the birds they could see outside. The confusion didn't lift, but the anxiety around it did.

These cloudier days don't require fixing. Your presence alone provides an anchor of stability. Sometimes the most helpful thing you can do is reduce stimulation - lower the television volume, speak more softly, or simply be quietly available.

Physical Factors That Make a Difference

Small physical discomforts can significantly impact how someone with dementia experiences their day. Poor sleep, constipation, hunger, or being too warm or cold can make confusion feel more overwhelming. While you might not be able to address these issues directly, recognizing their influence helps you respond with greater patience and understanding.

Kenneth learned to check basic comfort factors early in his visits. A glass of water, adjusting the thermostat, or suggesting a light snack often improved the entire afternoon's experience.

Embracing the Unpredictability

Instead of viewing this variability as a challenge, you can learn to see it as part of the natural human experience. We all have better days and worse days, though dementia makes these fluctuations more pronounced.

This understanding prepares you for the deeper insights we'll explore in the next chapter about why your presence matters so much, regardless of what kind of day you encounter.

Finding Magic in Mundane Moments

Perhaps the biggest adjustment for new helpers is realizing that meaningful help often looks remarkably ordinary. There are no dramatic breakthroughs or profound moments of connection - just small, steady acts of presence and care.

What Helpful Really Looks Like

During your time helping, you'll discover that:

- Success might look like a peaceful afternoon where nothing remarkable happens
- Helpful moments often involve simple activities: sharing a meal, watching television together, or sitting in comfortable silence
- Your presence itself provides comfort and security, even when it doesn't feel particularly significant to you
- The most valuable gift you offer is consistency and calm acceptance

This ordinariness is actually a gift. It means you don't need special skills or dramatic gestures to be helpful. You just need to show up with patience and kindness.

Dorothy had expected that helping her neighbor would involve managing constant confusion or providing complex care. Instead, she found herself spending most of their time together looking through old magazines and commenting on the pictures. Her neighbor enjoyed pointing out fashions she remembered and sharing brief stories about similar dresses she'd owned. It felt almost too simple to be helpful. Still, Dorothy could see how much her neighbor looked forward to these ordinary moments of connection.

The Power of Unremarkable Afternoons

Many helpers worry that their visits aren't meaningful because nothing dramatic occurs. This misses the profound value of stability and routine connection. When someone's world feels uncertain due to memory changes, your predictable presence becomes an anchor of normalcy.

Vincent discovered this during his weekly Saturday visits with his father-in-law. They rarely did anything exciting - usually just sat on the porch talking about the weather and watching cars go by. Vincent initially felt guilty that he wasn't providing more stimulating activities. Then he noticed how his father-in-law began mentioning these visits to others during the week, clearly treasuring the reliable rhythm of their time together.

Recognizing Success in Small Moments

Success in dementia help isn't measured by memory improvement or behavioral changes. Instead, look for:

- Moments of contentment and relaxation
- Smiles, laughter, or signs of enjoyment
- Reduced anxiety or agitation during your visit
- Peaceful transitions when you arrive or leave

These subtle indicators tell you that your presence is making a real difference, even when it doesn't feel dramatic to you.

The Ripple Effect You Create

Your visits create benefits that extend far beyond the hours you spend together. Regular helpers provide primary caregivers with essential breaks, reducing their stress and burnout. This improved caregiver wellbeing directly benefits the person with dementia.

Martha learned this when the primary caregiver thanked her for the weekly respite her visits provided. Those few hours allowed the caregiver to run errands, take a shower, or simply rest without worry. The peace of mind created by reliable help strengthened the entire care situation.

Recap of Key Points

Dementia in daily life is far more ordinary and manageable than most people expect. Rather than constant crisis or dramatic confusion, you're likely to encounter someone who's fundamentally still themselves, just with some differences in how they process information or remember details. Each visit may feel different depending on various factors, but your role remains consistent: to provide calm, patient presence. The most helpful thing you can do is let go of expectations about what help should look like and embrace the simple, human moments of connection that actually matter most.

Action Steps

Before your first visit, take a moment to adjust your expectations. Instead of preparing for dramatic challenges, prepare for ordinary moments that might unfold at a different pace than usual. Remind yourself that repetitive questions, small confusions, or quiet periods aren't problems you need to solve - they're simply part of the experience. Most importantly, remember that your calm presence is valuable even when it doesn't feel particularly significant to you.

Now that you understand what dementia actually looks like in daily life, you might still be wondering whether your help truly makes a difference. In the next chapter, we'll explore why helpers matter far more than they often realize - and how even small acts of presence create ripples of support that extend well beyond the time you spend together.

Why Your Help Matters More Than You Realize

Small Acts, Big System Wins

When you step in to help someone with dementia, you're not just helping that one person for that one moment. You're supporting an entire network of care that extends far beyond what you can see. Think of it like dropping a stone into still water - the ripples spread outward in ways you might never fully realize.

Your presence creates multiple layers of support:

· The primary caregiver gets a break without worry, knowing their loved one is in caring hands

· The person with dementia experiences continuity of care and familiar faces, which reduces anxiety and confusion

· Family members feel supported and less isolated, knowing they're not carrying the burden alone

Quinn had been caring for her husband with early-stage dementia for two years when her neighbor offered to sit with him for a few hours each Thursday morning. At first, Quinn felt guilty about leaving - what if something went wrong? But those Thursday mornings became her lifeline. She could grocery shop without rushing, have coffee with a friend, or simply sit in her car and breathe.

More importantly, her husband began looking forward to his neighbor's visits. The familiar face and gentle conversation became a highlight of his week. What started as a simple offer to help created a ripple effect: Quinn felt less overwhelmed, her husband felt more socially connected, and their adult children worried less about their parents because they knew support was in place.

The Caregiver Crisis Hidden in Plain Sight

Primary caregivers are burning out at alarming rates. Statistics tell us that family caregivers experience depression at twice the rate of the general population. They're more likely to have health problems themselves. Many give up jobs, drain savings, and sacrifice their own well-being.

When you offer to help, you're not just being nice.

You're potentially saving someone from complete exhaustion.

Consider what happens when primary caregivers reach their breaking point. The person with dementia often ends up in emergency situations - hospital visits, rushed placement decisions, or care from stressed, overwhelmed family members who can barely function themselves. Your few hours of support can prevent these crisis moments from happening.

Christian learned this firsthand when his sister called him in tears. She'd been caring for their mother with mid-stage dementia for three years without significant help. She was having chest pains, couldn't sleep, and felt like she was drowning. Christian started coming over every Saturday morning for four hours. His sister used that time to see her doctor, catch up on sleep, and slowly rebuild her strength. Their mother stayed in familiar surroundings longer because the care system became sustainable.

Why Familiar Faces Matter

As we discussed in Chapter 1, dementia affects how people process and remember information. New faces can be confusing or frightening. But when you become a regular helper, something beautiful happens. You become part of their world in a way that feels safe and predictable.

Regular helpers often notice things that others miss:

- Changes in mood or behavior patterns
- Physical symptoms that need attention
- Preferences and dislikes that make daily care smoother
- Small joys that bring comfort

Your consistent presence creates stability in a world that often feels chaotic and unpredictable for someone with dementia. This stability has real medical benefits - lower stress hormones, better sleep patterns, and fewer behavioral challenges.

Building Community Around Care

When you help regularly, you're modeling something powerful for others. Friends, neighbors, and church members see that helping with dementia care isn't impossible or scary. They see you managing it, and they begin to think maybe they could help too.

This creates expanding circles of support that benefit everyone involved.

The Caregiver's Hidden Wish List

Primary caregivers often struggle to articulate what they need most. It's rarely about grand gestures or complex assistance. Instead, it's about three fundamental things that restore their sense of balance and hope: relief from constant vigilance, a return to normalcy, and the comfort of knowing their loved one has other caring people in their life.

Derek cared for his mother, who lived with mid-stage dementia in his home. His sister lived across the country and felt helpless as she watched her brother shoulder everything alone. During her visits, she noticed he never seemed to fully relax, even when she was there helping. One evening, she suggested he go to his weekly poker game - something he'd given up months earlier. "But what if Mom gets confused? What if she asks for me?" he worried. His sister assured him she would handle whatever came up.

That night, for the first time in months, Derek laughed with his friends, forgot about dementia for a few hours, and returned home refreshed. His mother had spent the evening looking through old photo albums with her daughter, perfectly content. Derek realized he'd been so focused on being indispensable that he'd forgotten the value of simply being human.

What Caregivers Really Want But Can't Ask For

Most primary caregivers have learned to minimize their needs. They've adapted to a reality in which their wants seem selfish compared to their loved one's needs. But beneath the surface, they're longing for specific types of support that you can easily provide.

Permission to be imperfect: Caregivers carry enormous guilt about not doing enough, not being patient enough, not knowing enough. When you step in without judgment and handle situations differently than they would, you give them permission to realize there's no single "right" way to provide care.

Adult conversation and connection: As we explored in Chapter 1, dementia dramatically changes communication patterns. Caregivers often go days without having any meaningful conversations. Your presence helps them feel like themselves again.

The gift of ordinary moments: Simple activities like showering without rushing, reading a book, or having a phone conversation become luxuries. These aren't selfish desires - they're basic human needs that fuel the ability to continue caregiving long-term.

The Respite They Don't Think They Deserve

Many caregivers resist accepting help because they believe they should be able to handle everything themselves. This thinking stems from several sources: societal expectations, family guilt, and the gradual increase in the demands of dementia care. What starts as occasional assistance grows into round-the-clock responsibility so slowly that caregivers don't realize how much they've taken on.

Olivia had been caring for her husband with early-stage dementia for eighteen months when her church friend offered to visit weekly. Olivia initially said no - her husband was "still pretty good" and didn't need watching. Her friend persisted gently, suggesting she just wanted to visit and keep Olivia company. During these visits, Olivia discovered something surprising: having another person present changed the entire dynamic. She could focus on her husband's needs without feeling like the sole source of entertainment and engagement. She could step into the kitchen to prepare dinner without worry. Most importantly, she remembered what it felt like to share the emotional load with someone who cared.

Breaking the Isolation Cycle

Dementia caregiving creates a unique form of isolation. Unlike other health conditions where friends rally with meals and visits, dementia often drives people away. The unpredictable behaviors, communication challenges, and sheer length of the disease process cause many relationships to fade.

Your consistent presence breaks this pattern.

When you show up regularly and handle whatever the day brings, you demonstrate that dementia doesn't have to mean social death. Other friends and family members see your example and often find the courage to reengage.

One Hour Changes Everything

It's easy to underestimate the power of simply being present with someone who has dementia. You might think that because you're not providing medical care or solving problems, your contribution isn't significant. But calm, unhurried presence is often exactly what's needed most.

Your relaxed energy helps create an atmosphere of safety and peace. Consistent, gentle interaction provides a social connection that many people with dementia lack. Even brief periods of engagement can improve mood and reduce agitation for hours afterward.

Uma volunteered to visit her elderly neighbor once a week after learning he had dementia and his daughter was struggling to manage visits from three hours away. She worried she wasn't doing enough - they mostly just sat together, sometimes in comfortable silence, sometimes chatting about the weather or the birds at his feeder. She felt awkward when he repeated the same stories or forgot her name mid-conversation.

But his daughter noticed remarkable changes. On the days after Uma's visits, her father seemed calmer on their phone calls. He mentioned "the nice lady who comes to see me" and seemed to carry that warmth through the week. What felt like "just sitting together" to Uma was providing an essential human connection that rippled through his entire week.

The Science Behind Simple Presence

Research shows that people with dementia retain emotional memories even when factual memories fade. This means they might not remember your name or what you talked about, but they remember feeling cared for, safe, and valued. As we discussed in Chapter 1, the brain changes that come with dementia don't eliminate the fundamental human need for connection and companionship.

Your presence provides several measurable benefits:

- Reduced cortisol levels from stress relief
- Improved sleep patterns from feeling secure
- Better appetite from social dining experiences
- Decreased behavioral challenges from feeling less isolated

What Happens in That First Hour

When you first arrive, the person with dementia might seem uncertain or confused about who you are. This is completely normal and doesn't mean your visit isn't welcome or helpful. Give them time to adjust to your presence without pressure to remember you or engage in complex conversation.

Start with simple, non-threatening activities:

- Looking through photo albums together
- Listening to familiar music
- Sitting by a window and commenting on what you see outside
- Gentle activities like folding laundry or sorting items

Graham discovered this during his first visit with his church member's father. He arrived with elaborate plans for activities and conversation topics, but the older man seemed overwhelmed and agitated. Graham shifted his approach, simply sitting quietly and commenting occasionally on the birds outside the window. Within twenty minutes, his friend relaxed and began pointing out different birds he recognized. They spent the rest of the hour in peaceful companionship, and Graham learned that sometimes the best plans are no plans at all.

The Ripple Effect of Regular Visits

When you commit to regular visits, even short ones, you become part of the person's routine and environment, providing ongoing benefits. They begin to anticipate your visits, even if they can't articulate why Tuesday feels different or special.

Primary caregivers often report that their loved ones have better days overall when regular visitors are part of their schedule. The consistency provides structure and something to look forward to, both crucial elements for managing dementia symptoms.

Setting Up Others for Success

Your example of successful, low-pressure visits often encourages other friends and family members to try helping too. When they see that you're managing visits without drama or crisis, they realize it might not be as scary or difficult as they imagined.

This creates a support network that benefits everyone involved.

The key is to start simple and let the relationship develop naturally, as we'll explore in the next chapter about releasing the fear of doing things wrong.

You're the Energy They've Been Missing

Primary caregivers, no matter how loving and dedicated, inevitably experience fatigue, frustration, and emotional depletion. When you step in with fresh energy and perspective, you offer something precious that they simply cannot generate for themselves after months or years of intensive caregiving.

Your enthusiasm for simple activities can reignite joy that daily caregiving may have dimmed. You bring new conversation topics and a different personality, providing stimulating variety. Your calm presence can break cycles of tension or routine that may have developed between the primary caregiver and their loved one.

Cole noticed his grandmother seemed increasingly withdrawn during his weekly visits to help his aunt, who was her primary caregiver. His aunt was devoted but exhausted, and their interactions had become focused on tasks - medications, meals, personal care. During one visit, Cole simply sat with his grandmother and asked about her childhood. To his surprise, she became animated, sharing stories he'd never heard. His aunt stood in the doorway, tears in her eyes. "I haven't seen her this engaged in months," she whispered.

Cole realized that while his aunt provided excellent care, she was too tired and too close to the daily struggles to access the playful, curious energy that could still reach his grandmother. His fresh perspective and genuine interest unlocked a part of her that had seemed lost.

The Gift of a Different Perspective

As we explored in Chapter 1, dementia affects each person uniquely, and their needs change throughout the day and across different stages. What works for the primary caregiver might not be the only approach that brings comfort or engagement. Your different personality, communication style, and interests offer new pathways to connection.

Consider these fresh approaches you might naturally bring:

- Different music preferences that spark unexpected memories
- Varied conversation topics based on your own experiences and interests
- Alternative ways of approaching daily activities that feel less routine
- A different pace or energy level that matches their needs in the moment

Breaking the Caregiver Burnout Cycle

Primary caregivers often develop tunnel vision from the intensity of their role. They become so focused on safety, medical needs, and daily tasks that they lose sight of the person beyond the diagnosis. This isn't their fault - it's a natural response to overwhelming responsibility.

Your presence can interrupt this cycle.

When you arrive without the weight of daily caregiving responsibilities, you can see and respond to aspects of their personality that may have become buried under routine care. You might notice their sense of humor, their love of certain topics, or their enjoyment of specific activities that the primary caregiver has forgotten or feels too tired to pursue.

The Energy Exchange Effect

Dementia care involves enormous emotional labor. Primary caregivers constantly monitor, anticipate, redirect, and manage challenging situations. This depletes their emotional reserves and can create a tense or vigilant atmosphere, even when they're trying to be positive.

Your fresh energy changes the entire dynamic of the environment. People with dementia are highly sensitive to the emotional atmosphere around them, as we discussed in Chapter 1. When you bring calm, unhurried presence without the underlying stress of constant responsibility, they respond to that difference.

Fiona discovered this when she started visiting her church friend's husband once a week. The primary caregiver had mentioned that afternoons were particularly difficult - he became agitated and restless. During Fiona's first visit, she expected challenges but found him surprisingly peaceful. She later realized that her relaxed attitude, combined with her not being responsible for his overall well-being, created an energy he found soothing.

Setting Everyone Up for Success

Your role as a supportive visitor creates benefits for everyone involved. The person with dementia experiences variety and stimulation. The primary caregiver gets relief and perspective. You gain meaningful connections and the satisfaction of making a real difference.

The key is understanding that you're not replacing the primary caregiver or competing with them.

You're complementing their care with something they cannot provide for themselves - fresh perspective, renewed energy, and the gift of seeing their loved one through completely different eyes.

Letting Go of the Fear of "Doing It Wrong"

Ready Never Comes, Help Anyway

DIANA HAD BEEN MEANING to visit her neighbor for three months. She'd watched through her kitchen window as the daily care worker arrived each morning, and she'd noticed how tired the neighbor's daughter looked when she stopped by after work. "I should offer to help," she thought repeatedly. But then the questions would start: What if I say something that upsets her? What if she asks me something I don't know how to answer? What if I make her condition worse somehow? Three months turned into six, and the help never materialized - not because she didn't care, but because she was waiting to feel confident enough to be perfect.

The perfectionism trap is perhaps the biggest barrier between willing helpers and people who need support. It convinces us that we must be fully prepared, completely knowledgeable, and entirely confident before we can be useful. This trap is particularly cruel because it disguises fear as responsibility, making us believe we're being careful when we're actually being paralyzed.

The myth of readiness: There is no moment when you'll suddenly feel "ready enough" to help someone with dementia. Readiness comes through gentle experience, not through endless preparation.

Competence versus presence: Professional caregivers develop competence through training and repetition, but what most people with dementia need from friends and family is presence - something that requires no special training at all.

The cost of waiting: Every day spent waiting to feel more prepared is a day when help isn't offered, and connections aren't made. The person you want to help still needs support, while you feel inadequate.

Isaac finally decided to visit his uncle after his cousin mentioned feeling overwhelmed. He arrived with no plan except to "see how things were going." His uncle didn't remember his name that day, but they spent two hours looking through old photographs together. Isaac later realized he'd been so focused on what he didn't know about dementia that he'd forgotten what he did know about his uncle - his love of baseball, his tendency to tell the same three stories, his preference for sitting by the window.

The visit wasn't perfect, but it was exactly what both of them needed.

Remember from Chapter 2 how your presence alone provides relief for exhausted caregivers and meaningful connection for people with dementia. That impact doesn't require perfection. It requires showing up with kindness and flexibility, two qualities you already possess.

Your fear of "doing it wrong" often centers around specific worries that seem reasonable on the surface but dissolve when examined closely. What if they don't remember me? Memory loss doesn't erase the comfort that comes from familiar faces and gentle voices. What if I don't know what to say? Sometimes the best conversations happen when we stop trying to fill every silence with words. What if they get confused or upset? Confusion and emotional moments are part of dementia, not something you cause by being present.

The truth is simpler than your anxious mind suggests.

You cannot break someone with dementia by being imperfect. You cannot make the patient's condition worse by caring awkwardly. You cannot ruin everything by not knowing all the answers.

But you can miss opportunities to connect by waiting for impossible certainty.

As we move into Chapter 4 and explore communication techniques, remember that the foundation of all helpful interaction is your willingness to be present, even in the face of uncertainty. The specific skills matter less than your genuine desire to connect and support. Start from that place of authentic care, and the rest will follow more naturally than you expect.

When Worry Meets Reality

Most people's fears about "doing it wrong" center around imagined catastrophes rather than actual risks. We picture ourselves saying something that causes lasting emotional damage, or accidentally triggering a medical emergency, or somehow making the dementia progression worse through our inexperience. These fears feel very real, but they rarely reflect what actually goes wrong when untrained helpers step in with good intentions.

Real concerns are typically about immediate safety and dignity - things like someone wandering away unsupervised, medication being given incorrectly, or a person being left in a dangerous situation. Imagined concerns tend to focus on social awkwardness, conversational mistakes, or not knowing the "right" way to handle confusion or repetition.

Safety versus comfort: Actual "wrong" usually involves physical safety (leaving someone alone who shouldn't be, ignoring signs of medical distress) rather than social discomfort (not knowing how to respond to a repeated question).

Temporary versus permanent: Most mistakes helpers worry about are temporary inconveniences - a moment of confusion, an awkward silence, a small disagreement - rather than lasting harm.

Intent matters: People with dementia are often remarkably good at sensing whether someone cares about them, even when that person doesn't know exactly what to do or say.

Uma was terrified she'd say something wrong when she agreed to stay with her friend's mother for an afternoon. She spent the first hour walking on eggshells, carefully measuring every word. Then Uma's friend's mother asked, for the fifth time, when her daughter would be home. Uma finally relaxed and said, "I'm not sure exactly, but she'll be back later today. Would you like some tea while we wait?" That simple, honest response worked better than any of her carefully rehearsed phrases. She realized that her friend's mother didn't need perfect answers - she needed someone who would respond kindly to her questions, however many times she asked them.

The gap between worry and reality becomes clearer when we examine what actually creates distress for people with dementia. Sharp tones, impatience, and dismissive responses cause more upset than confused answers or gentle honesty. Being ignored hurts more than being misunderstood. Feeling rushed creates more anxiety than taking time to figure things out together.

Building on what we learned in Chapter 2 about the profound impact of your presence, consider how your anxious energy affects the person you're trying to help. When you're tense about making mistakes, that tension transfers to them. When you're rigid about doing everything "correctly," you miss opportunities to be naturally responsive to their actual needs in the moment.

Frank discovered this during his first visit with his elderly neighbor. He'd prepared extensively, reading articles and watching videos about dementia care. But when he arrived, his neighbor wanted to show him the garden, not discuss current events as Frank had planned. His initial instinct was to redirect the conversation to something he felt more prepared for. Instead, he followed his neighbor outside. They spent an hour looking at tomato plants and talking about summer weather. Later, Frank realized that the most helpful thing he'd done was abandon his script and follow his neighbor's lead.

Your biggest mistake isn't saying the wrong thing or handling confusion imperfectly.

Your biggest mistake is letting fear keep you away entirely.

The person who needs support doesn't need your perfection - they need your willingness to be present through the imperfect moments. As we move into Chapter 4 and explore specific communication approaches, remember that the foundation of all helpful interaction is your genuine desire to connect, not your technical expertise.

Awkward Moments Are Growth Opportunities

Awkwardness is not failure - it's simply what happens when humans interact with other humans in unfamiliar circumstances. When you're helping someone with dementia, there will be moments when you don't know what to say, when conversations don't make complete sense, when you feel uncertain about how to respond. These moments feel much more significant to you than they do to the person you're helping.

People with dementia are often more forgiving of social awkwardness than we might expect. They may not remember the specific details of an uncomfortable moment. Still, they will retain the general feeling of whether someone was kind to them. Your nervousness about saying the wrong thing matters far less than your willingness to stay present and engaged.

Awkward doesn't mean harmful: Feeling uncertain about how to respond to confusion or repetition is normal and doesn't cause distress to the person with dementia.

Recovery is always possible: If a conversation goes sideways or a moment feels uncomfortable, you can always redirect gently, change the subject, or simply sit quietly together.

Perfection isn't expected: The people who love and care for someone with dementia aren't expecting you to be flawless - they're grateful that you're willing to help at all.

Drew agreed to take his neighbor to a doctor's appointment, confident that this straightforward task would be manageable. But in the waiting room, his neighbor began talking loudly about very personal medical details, seemingly unaware that others could hear. Drew felt mortified and wasn't sure whether to try to quiet him or just pretend it wasn't happening. He chose to lean in and respond quietly, hoping his neighbor would match his lower volume. It worked partially - the conversation continued, but more quietly. Later, Drew realized that his embarrassment had been much more intense than his neighbor's. The appointment went fine, and his neighbor thanked him warmly for the ride. What had felt like a social disaster to Drew had simply been an ordinary moment to someone whose relationship with social conventions had changed.

These awkward moments actually serve as valuable learning experiences. Each one teaches you something about dementia, about the specific person you're helping, and about your own assumptions and reactions. The grandmother who insists you're her long-lost cousin isn't testing your honesty - she's showing you how her brain is working that day. The friend who asks the same question repeatedly isn't questioning your previous answers - he's demonstrating how his memory is affected.

Consider how these moments connect to what we discussed in Chapter 2 about your meaningful impact. Your presence during awkward moments - your willingness to stay engaged even when things don't go according to plan - provides exactly the kind of patient, accepting interaction that exhausted caregivers desperately need breaks from and that people with dementia benefit from experiencing.

Olivia learned this during her first afternoon helping with her church friend's mother. She'd prepared conversation topics and brought photo albums. Still, her friend's mother seemed confused and kept calling her by the wrong name. Olivia spent the first hour gently correcting the mistake, feeling increasingly frustrated. Finally, she decided to respond to the name her friend's mother was using. The conversation immediately became more relaxed and enjoyable. Her friend's mother began sharing stories and laughing, apparently comfortable now that Olivia had stopped fighting the confusion.

The lesson wasn't about giving up accuracy - it was about recognizing when flexibility serves connection better than correctness.

As we move forward to explore specific communication techniques in Chapter 4, remember that your willingness to navigate awkward moments with grace and humor is itself a valuable skill. The specific words matter less than your genuine care and adaptability.

When to Call in the Experts

One of the biggest fears that keeps people from helping is not knowing when a situation requires professional intervention. This fear is understandable, but it often leads to overcaution that prevents anyone from offering help. The truth is that most situations requiring professional help are quite obvious - they involve immediate medical concerns, safety risks, or behaviors that seem dangerous rather than simply unusual.

Understanding the difference between "I should call someone" situations and "this is just different from what I'm used to" situations can free you to be helpful in the vast majority of circumstances. Most of the time, your role is simply to provide companionship and maintain a calm environment, not to make medical or safety decisions.

Clear warning signs: Situations requiring immediate professional help usually involve obvious medical distress, safety dangers (like someone trying to leave and getting lost), or extreme agitation that you can't calm.

When in doubt, ask: If you're unsure whether something requires professional attention, it's always appropriate to call the primary caregiver or a medical professional for guidance.

Most moments are manageable: The vast majority of your time helping someone with dementia will involve ordinary moments - conversation, simple activities, routine tasks - that don't require any special expertise.

Sophia was staying with her aunt for the weekend when her aunt became convinced that strangers were in the house and began repeatedly checking all the locks. Sophia's first instinct was to call her aunt's daughter immediately, worried that this was a sign of something seriously wrong. Instead, she stayed calm and asked her aunt if she'd like some company while checking the locks. They walked through the house together, and Sophia casually mentioned how secure everything looked. After about twenty minutes, her aunt seemed to forget about the concern and asked if they could watch television together. Sophia realized that what had felt like a crisis requiring intervention was actually just a moment of anxiety that passed naturally. She did mention it to her cousin later, but as information rather than an emergency. Her cousin thanked her for staying calm and explained that these episodes happened occasionally but usually resolved on their own when someone responded matter-of-factly rather than with alarm.

Recap of Key Points

The fear of "doing it wrong" is often more paralyzing than helpful, preventing well-meaning people from offering support that could make a real difference. Most of our fears about helping someone with dementia are based on imagined disasters rather than realistic risks. Perfectionism keeps us waiting for a readiness that never comes, while the people we want to help continue to need the presence and companionship we could offer right now.

Actual mistakes in dementia care usually involve clear safety or medical concerns, not the social awkwardness or conversational uncertainty that most helpers worry about. Awkward moments are normal parts of human interaction and don't constitute failure or harm. People with dementia are often more forgiving of our imperfections than we are, and they're usually more interested in our kindness than our competence.

Action Steps

· Identify one specific fear you have about helping someone with dementia and ask yourself: "Is this about safety, or is this about my own discomfort?"

· Think of a time when someone was patient with your own confusion or mistakes. Remember how their kindness mattered more than their perfect responses

· Consider one small way you could offer help this week - a phone call, a short visit, or offering to accompany someone on an errand - without waiting to feel completely prepared

Now that we've addressed the fears that often prevent people from helping, it's time to focus on what actually does help. The next chapter will explore communication approaches that create calm and connection, showing you that effective communication with someone who has dementia is less about finding perfect words and more about creating a sense of safety and understanding.

This is common. Your nervousness about helping doesn't mean you're not ready - it means you care enough to want to do well.

Communication That Soothes

Your Voice Speaks Louder Than Words

YOUR TONE OF VOICE carries more weight than the actual words you choose when communicating with someone living with dementia. A gentle, unhurried tone can transform even the most mundane conversation into something that feels safe and reassuring.

After reading Chapter 3 about letting go of fear, you might still wonder exactly how to speak in ways that create comfort rather than confusion. The answer lies not in memorizing perfect phrases, but in adjusting how you deliver your words.

The Power of Tone

Mia was helping her neighbor for the afternoon when she noticed something remarkable. Every time she asked a question in her usual brisk tone, her neighbor looked confused and slightly anxious. But when Mia slowed down and softened her voice - asking the same question about whether she'd like some tea - her neighbor's face relaxed immediately, and she responded with a smile.

The words were identical. The delivery made all the difference.

Research shows that people with dementia often retain their ability to read emotional cues in voices long after language processing becomes difficult. Your tone communicates safety or stress, patience or pressure, love or frustration. They hear your heart through your voice.

Simple Voice Adjustments That Work

- Speak slowly and clearly without sounding patronizing or childlike
- Keep your voice at a lower pitch and softer volume than usual conversation
- Allow natural pauses between sentences to give processing time

Think of how you might speak to a close friend who's had a long, difficult day. That gentle, caring tone is exactly what works best.

Beyond Words: What Your Voice Conveys

When Harrison first started visiting his uncle, he brought his usual energetic personality into every conversation. His uncle seemed overwhelmed and often retreated to his room. After adjusting his approach - speaking more quietly and leaving space between thoughts - his uncle began engaging more and even sharing old stories.

Your voice tells the person with dementia whether this interaction will be pleasant or stressful. A rushed, impatient tone signals danger to their nervous system. A calm, steady voice signals safety.

Practical Voice Techniques

Start each conversation with a warm greeting that includes their name. This helps orient them to who you are and that you're glad to see them. Instead of jumping into questions or tasks, spend a moment simply being present with them.

Use shorter sentences with one main idea each. Rather than saying, "Would you like some water, or maybe tea, or we could get you some juice if you prefer that instead," try, "Would you like some water?" Wait for their response. Then offer another option if needed.

When Words Don't Come Easily

Sometimes the person you're helping will struggle to find words or lose their train of thought mid-sentence. Your voice becomes even more important during these moments. A gentle "take your time" or "that's okay" can prevent frustration from building.

Mia learned to fill comfortable silences with soft observations like "the birds sound lovely today" or "this sunshine feels nice." These simple comments took pressure off the conversation while maintaining connection.

Setting Up Success for Chapter 5

As you practice these voice techniques, you'll notice that communication becomes less about perfect words and more about creating emotional safety. This foundation becomes crucial when handling repetitive questions and confusion - topics we'll explore in Chapter 5. When your voice already signals calm and patience, repetitive conversations feel less overwhelming for everyone involved.

Your voice is a gift you bring to every interaction. Use it wisely.

The Power of Silence

Sometimes the most soothing communication happens without words at all. Your body language, facial expressions, and comfort with quiet moments often communicate more effectively than any conversation could.

Building on what you learned in Chapter 3 about releasing the fear of doing it wrong, you might still feel pressure to keep conversations going or worry when silence stretches between you and the person you're helping. This anxiety about quiet moments can actually create more stress for everyone involved.

When Your Presence Speaks Volumes

Lucas discovered this during his first weekend helping his uncle. After struggling through several confusing conversations, he simply sat quietly beside his uncle on the porch. They watched the birds together for nearly an hour, with Lucas occasionally pointing out a cardinal or nodding when his uncle made a comment. Later, his aunt mentioned it was the most peaceful her husband had seemed in weeks.

The magic happened in the silence, not the words.

People with dementia often feel overwhelmed by too much verbal input. Your calm presence can provide the emotional regulation they need more than any specific conversation topic. When you're comfortable with quiet, they can relax too.

Your Body Speaks First

Before you say a single word, your body language has already started the conversation. Tense shoulders, hurried movements, or an anxious expression can trigger stress responses. But relaxed posture, gentle movements, and a peaceful face create immediate comfort.

Key Body Language Basics:

- Maintain a relaxed, open body posture and gentle facial expressions
- Use simple gestures like offering your arm or pointing to guide rather than lengthy explanations
- Move slowly and deliberately rather than rushing through tasks

Sarah learned this when helping her neighbor get ready for a doctor's appointment. Initially, she rushed around gathering items while rattling off instructions. Her neighbor became agitated and confused. When Sarah slowed down, made eye contact, and used simple pointing gestures to indicate each item they needed, the process became smooth and calm.

The Gift of Comfortable Silence

Many helpers feel they must fill every moment with chatter to avoid awkwardness. This pressure often creates the opposite effect. Constant talking can overwhelm someone whose brain is already working hard to process information.

Embrace comfortable silence instead of feeling pressured to fill every moment with talk.

Think of silence as space for connection rather than emptiness to fill. During quiet moments, you might both notice a beautiful sunset, listen to familiar music, or simply enjoy each other's company. These shared experiences often create deeper bonds than forced conversation.

Simple Gestures That Guide

When words feel complicated, gentle gestures become incredibly helpful. A warm smile, an outstretched hand, or a soft touch on the shoulder can communicate welcome, assistance, or comfort more clearly than verbal explanations.

Lucas discovered that pointing to items while saying their names helped his father navigate daily tasks more easily than verbal directions alone. "Here's your coffee," while gesturing toward the cup, worked better than explaining where he'd placed it.

Reading Their Silent Cues

Just as your nonverbal communication matters, learning to read their body language helps you respond appropriately. Fidgeting might indicate discomfort or restlessness. Withdrawn posture could signal overstimulation or fatigue. A relaxed face and open posture show contentment.

Preparing for What's Ahead

As you become more comfortable with silent communication, you'll find it easier to handle the repetitive questions and moments of confusion we'll explore in Chapter 5. When you're not relying solely on words to connect, repetition becomes less frustrating, and confusion feels more manageable.

Your peaceful presence is a powerful gift. Trust it.

Step Into Their World Gently

One of the most challenging aspects of communication is resisting the natural impulse to correct misunderstandings or redirect confused thinking. Instead of fighting their reality, gently entering it creates a connection rather than conflict.

This approach builds directly on the fear-releasing principles from Chapter 3, where you learned that being "right" matters less than being helpful. Now you can take that insight deeper into actual conversations.

Why Corrections Create Conflict

When someone with dementia expresses confusion about time, place, or people, your instinct might be to gently correct them. This feels helpful and caring. But corrections often trigger frustration, embarrassment, or even anger because you're essentially telling them their brain is wrong.

Consider what that feels like. Imagine confidently stating something you believe to be true, only to have someone correct you repeatedly throughout the day.

It's exhausting and demoralizing.

Entering Their Reality Instead

When Morgan was visiting her grandmother, the older woman insisted that she pick up her children from school, who were now adults in their fifties. Instead of explaining this wasn't necessary, Morgan said, "You're such a caring mother. Your children are lucky to have you." Her grandmother smiled and relaxed, the urgency fading as she felt heard and valued.

This response acknowledged the emotional truth behind the confusion. The grandmother wasn't really confused about her children's ages. She was expressing her deep identity as a caring mother and her concern for their well-being.

Practical Response Techniques

Acknowledge their feelings and experiences without necessarily agreeing with factual details. This validates their emotional reality while avoiding arguments about facts that don't really matter in the moment.

Use phrases like:

- "That sounds important."
- "Tell me more about that."
- "You really care about them."
- "That must be on your mind."

These responses show respect for their concerns without getting tangled up in timeline corrections or reality checks that serve no helpful purpose.

Focus on Emotion, Not Facts

When Jonathan visited his uncle, the older man frequently talked about needing to get home to his wife, who had passed away years earlier. Instead of reminding him about his wife's death, Jonathan learned to say, "You miss her" or "She sounds wonderful. Tell me about her." These conversations became opportunities to share loving memories rather than painful reminders of loss.

Focus on the emotion behind their words rather than the literal accuracy.

The person isn't usually seeking factual information. They're expressing feelings, concerns, or memories that matter to them. When you respond to those deeper needs, communication becomes meaningful rather than frustrating.

When Gentle Redirection Helps

Sometimes you can gently guide without direct correction. If someone asks about going to work even though that person has been retired for decades, you might say, "What did you like best about your job?" This honors their work identity while naturally shifting the conversation to reminiscence rather than current obligations.

Preparing for Repetition

As you practice entering their world more gently, you'll find these same conversations happening again and again. The person might ask about those school children every day or express the same concerns multiple times within an hour. Chapter 5 will show you how to handle this repetition with the same grace you're developing here, using the communication foundation you're building now.

Your willingness to step into their reality, even briefly, creates moments of genuine connection in a world that often feels confusing and corrective.

Words That Soothe Instead of Scramble

Having a mental toolkit of gentle, non-confrontational responses can help you navigate difficult moments without escalating confusion or distress. These phrases redirect without dismissing and validate without necessarily agreeing.

Building on your growing confidence from Chapter 3 about releasing the fear of doing it wrong, you now need specific language tools that work consistently. The right words can transform tense moments into opportunities for connection.

The Magic of Validation

Thomas learned the power of simple responses when his neighbor asked him fifteen times in one afternoon where her husband was. Instead of repeatedly explaining that her husband had passed away years ago, he began responding with, "He must be very special to you. Tell me about him." This shifted her focus from anxiety about his location to pleasant memories, and the repetitive questioning naturally faded.

The key was validation without false information. Thomas didn't lie about the husband's whereabouts, but he acknowledged the love and concern behind the question.

Calming Phrases for Anxious Moments

When someone with dementia feels frightened or disoriented, certain phrases can provide immediate comfort:

Use reassuring phrases like:

- "You're safe here."
- "I'm here with you."
- "Everything is okay right now."
- "You're doing fine."

These statements focus on the present moment and provide emotional anchoring when their world feels unstable. The person might not remember why they felt scared, but they'll remember feeling reassured.

Responding to Repetitive Questions

Instead of showing frustration when the same question comes up repeatedly, try these approaches:

Respond to repetitive questions with patience:

- "That's a good question."
- "I can see why you're wondering about that."
- "You're thinking about important things."
- "Let me think about that with you."

Sarah discovered that when her grandmother asked repeatedly about her purse, responding with "Your purse is important to you" led to stories about special occasions when she'd carried it. The anxiety about the missing purse gave way to pleasant reminiscing.

Gentle Redirection Instead of Refusal

Rather than using words that create resistance, offer alternatives that feel collaborative:

Offer gentle alternatives:

· "Let's sit here for a moment" instead of "No, you can't go there."

· "How about we try this," instead of "That's wrong."

· "I have an idea" instead of "You need to stop that."

· "Let's do this together" instead of "You can't do that alone."

Words That Build Instead of Block

Certain words naturally create cooperation while others trigger defensive responses. Notice the difference between "You forgot" and "Let me remind you." Both communicate the same information, but one feels accusatory while the other feels helpful.

Replace blocking language with building language:

· Instead of "Don't worry," try "You're safe."

· Instead of "You're confused," try "That's hard to remember."

· Instead of "That's not right," try "I see it differently."

Creating Your Personal Phrase Bank

As you spend time with someone, you'll notice which phrases work best for them. Some people respond well to gentle humor, while others prefer straightforward reassurance. Pay attention to what brings them peace and add those specific phrases to your personal toolkit.

Preparing for What's Coming

These communication tools become especially valuable when handling the repetitive conversations and moments of confusion that we'll explore thoroughly in Chapter 5. Having gentle responses ready helps you stay calm when the same questions come up repeatedly, laying a foundation for the grace you'll need in those challenging moments.

Your words have the power to soothe or scramble. Choose them wisely.

When Stories Unravel Before You

Listening with genuine interest to stories that may be fragmented, repetitive, or factually unclear is one of the greatest gifts you can offer. Your attentive presence validates their need to communicate and maintains their dignity as a person with something to say.

This skill builds naturally on everything you've learned so far about releasing perfectionist expectations and creating soothing communication environments. Now you can put those principles into practice during actual storytelling moments.

The Gift of Imperfect Stories

During her weekly visits, Lisa noticed that her aunt would tell the same story about her wedding day, but the details would change each time. Sometimes it was sunny, sometimes rainy. The dress was blue, then white, then her mother's dress. Instead of trying to establish the "correct" version, Lisa listened to each telling as if hearing it for the first time, asking about the flowers or the music. Her aunt's face would light up with each retelling, lost in the joy of sharing something precious.

The story's accuracy mattered far less than the connection it created.

Focus on Emotions and Themes

When someone with dementia tells stories, they're rarely seeking to provide you with factual information. They're sharing pieces of their identity, expressing feelings, or reconnecting with meaningful memories. The chronology might be scrambled, but the emotional core often remains intact.

Focus on the emotions and themes in their stories rather than on chronological accuracy. Listen for what made them proud, what brought them joy, or what worried them. These emotional truths matter more than whether the events happened in 1962 or 1972.

Engaging Without Correcting

Your questions can guide the conversation toward richer sharing without pointing out inconsistencies:

Ask gentle follow-up questions that show you're engaged:

- "How did that make you feel?"
- "What was that like?"
- "Who else was there?"
- "What did you enjoy most about that?"

These questions invite deeper reflection and demonstrate your genuine interest in their experience. They also help the person stay connected to positive emotions associated with their memories.

The Value of the Telling

Robert discovered that his father told the same war story differently each week during their Sunday visits. Rather than being concerned about the inconsistencies, Robert began to see that his father needed to process and repeatedly share this significant life experience. The act of telling helped his father maintain his identity as a veteran and connect with his son through shared storytelling.

Remember that telling the story often matters more than its coherence.

The person isn't usually trying to inform you about historical events. They're trying to connect with you, process their experiences, or maintain their sense of self through narrative.

When Stories Become Fragments

Sometimes stories don't have clear beginnings, middles, or ends. A person might start talking about their mother, then jump to their first job, and finally mention a dog from childhood. These fragmented narratives still deserve your attention and respect.

Follow their lead without trying to create logical connections. If they want to talk about three different decades in one conversation, let them. Your role isn't to organize their thoughts but to witness them with kindness.

Preparing for Repetition

As you become more comfortable with imperfect storytelling, you'll notice that certain stories or questions arise repeatedly throughout a single visit or across multiple visits. Chapter 5 will show you how to handle this repetition with the same grace you're developing here, using your growing communication skills to navigate those challenging moments without frustration.

Your willingness to listen honors their humanity and preserves their dignity as someone with experiences worth sharing.

Handling Repetition and Confusion With Grace

When Memory Forgets Your Face

THE SAME QUESTION COMES again. And again. And then once more, before you've even finished answering the previous time. This is the reality of dementia care that catches most helpers off guard - not the big, dramatic moments you might expect, but the gentle, persistent repetition that can slowly wear down your patience if you're not prepared for it.

Why Fighting Repetition Makes Everything Harder: Understanding the brain's new patterns

When someone has dementia, their brain creates new patterns of processing information that are completely different from what we consider normal. Fighting against these patterns by constantly correcting or explaining creates frustration for everyone involved, turning simple interactions into emotional battlegrounds that nobody wins.

Understanding that repetition isn't stubbornness or attention-seeking changes everything about how we respond.

The brain with dementia processes each repeated question as if it were the first time it was asked. Your loved one isn't trying to annoy you or test your patience. They genuinely don't remember asking the question moments before. This knowledge becomes your foundation for responding with grace instead of frustration.

Consider these key principles:

· Accept that repetition is communication, not a problem to solve

· Recognize that each repeated question feels fresh to them

· Understand that your calm response matters more than providing new information

Mia learned this lesson while helping her father-in-law during a weekend visit. He asked about his late wife's whereabouts every few minutes. Initially, Mia tried explaining that she had passed away two years ago. Each time, she watched him experience the grief anew. The repeated explanations weren't helping anyone - they were actually creating more pain.

Finally, she began responding with, "She's not here right now, but would you like to tell me about her?" The repetitive questions continued, but the emotional upheaval stopped. Mia realized she wasn't being dishonest - she was being kind. The questions weren't really about location; they were about connection and comfort.

This shift in understanding transforms how you approach moments of confusion. Instead of viewing repetition as something to fix, you start seeing it as an opportunity to offer reassurance and presence.

Practical responses that work:

When they ask where someone is, try redirecting to positive memories: "Tell me your favorite thing about her." When they worry about appointments or responsibilities, offer comfort: "Everything important is taken care of today."

Remember the communication techniques from Chapter 4 - your tone and body language matter more than your exact words. A gentle, patient response to the tenth repetition of the same question creates a sense of safety that fighting the repetition never could.

The confusion isn't going away, but your response can make each moment feel secure rather than stressful.

When they don't recognize you:

Perhaps the most heart-wrenching aspect of dementia progression is when familiar faces become strangers. This doesn't mean love has disappeared - it means the brain's filing system has changed. Your relationship continues even when recognition falters.

Don't take this personally.

Instead, focus on creating comfort in each interaction. Introduce yourself naturally: "Hi, I'm Mia, and I'm here to spend time with you today." Let them guide the interaction without forcing memories or connections they can't access.

This prepares you for the practical aspects of personal care we'll explore in Chapter 6, where these same principles of patience and acceptance become even more crucial.

When Answers Become Echoes

Repeated questions are often the most challenging aspect of helping someone with dementia, especially when you're volunteering for just an hour or an afternoon. The same inquiry surfaces every few minutes, testing your patience in ways you didn't expect when you offered to help. Understanding that each time they ask, it's genuinely the first time in their current awareness changes everything about how you respond.

Your response can either escalate their anxiety or provide the reassurance they're seeking.

The communication principles from Chapter 4 become crucial here - your tone, body language, and emotional state matter more than the actual words you choose. When facing repetitive questions, remember that fighting the pattern creates stress for everyone involved.

Key strategies that work:

- Answer with the same calm tone each time, as if it's the first time
- Keep responses short and reassuring rather than detailed
- Look for the emotion behind the question, not just the literal meaning

Adam was helping his aunt for an afternoon when she began asking every few minutes, "Did I take my medicine today?" Instead of getting frustrated or trying to convince her, Adam simply stated, "Your medicine is all taken care of." He kept a calm, reassuring tone each time.

By the third repetition, he noticed something important. His Aunt wasn't really asking about medicine - she was asking for reassurance that someone was looking after her health. His consistent, gentle response provided exactly what she needed, and eventually the questions naturally faded as her anxiety decreased.

This insight transforms how you handle repetitive conversations. Instead of viewing them as memory problems to correct, you start recognizing them as emotional needs seeking comfort.

Common repeated questions and what they really mean:

"Where is my husband?" often translates to "I feel alone and want connection."

When someone says, "When am I going home?" it usually means, "I want to feel safe and secure."

"What time is it?" frequently expresses "I feel lost and need structure."

Understanding these deeper meanings helps you respond to the heart of their concern rather than just the surface question. This approach aligns with the fear-reducing strategies we discussed in Chapter 3 - you're providing security instead of corrections.

Practical responses that soothe:

When someone repeatedly asks about a deceased spouse, avoid re-explaining the death each time. Instead, try: "Tell me about your favorite memory of him" or "He sounds like a wonderful person."

For questions about going home, consider: "You're safe here with me" or "Let's sit together for a while."

When they repeatedly ask about time, offer reassurance: "We have plenty of time to spend together today."

These responses honor their emotional state while maintaining the gentle, patient approach that creates trust. Your goal isn't to fix their memory - it's to provide comfort in the moment.

When confusion deepens:

Sometimes, repeated questions can deepen confusion about surroundings, people, or situations. This progression is normal and doesn't reflect your caregiving abilities. Stay anchored in the present moment, using the same calm presence that has been working.

Your consistent, peaceful responses create an environment where confusion feels less frightening. This foundation of trust becomes especially important when helping with more intimate tasks like personal care, which we'll explore in Chapter 6.

The key is maintaining your emotional balance while recognizing that each repeated interaction is an opportunity to offer comfort and connection, not a test of your patience or their memory.

Lost in Time's Shifting Maze

Time confusion is incredibly common in dementia and often causes distress for both the person and their helpers. When someone believes it's 1987 or thinks they need to pick up children who are now adults, your natural instinct might be to gently correct them and bring them back to reality. However, this approach often backfires, creating more anxiety and confusion than comfort.

The instinct to correct and reorient can actually increase confusion and agitation.

Understanding how dementia affects time perception helps you respond more effectively. The brain's ability to sequence events, understand cause and effect, and maintain awareness of the present moment becomes compromised. What feels like stubborn confusion to you is actually their brain doing its best with limited resources.

Building on the communication strategies from Chapter 4, your response to time confusion should prioritize emotional comfort over factual accuracy. This doesn't mean lying or being dishonest - it means choosing responses that reduce distress while honoring their current experience.

Effective approaches include:

· Avoid lengthy explanations about what day it actually is

· Respond to the feeling behind their time-related concerns

· Use phrases like "later" or "soon" instead of specific times when redirecting

Sarah was staying with her grandmother when the older woman became anxious about being late for work, work she had retired from fifteen years earlier. Sarah's first instinct was to explain about retirement and the current date, reminding her grandmother that she was now in her eighties and hadn't worked in years.

Instead, she remembered the principles from Chapter 3 about letting go of the need to always be "right."

"It's still early. Would you like some breakfast first?" Sarah said, acknowledging her grandmother's concern without challenging reality. This simple response validated the underlying anxiety about responsibility while gently redirecting toward a pleasant activity.

They spent a pleasant morning together, and the work anxiety naturally faded as they settled into familiar morning routines. Sarah learned that meeting someone where they are emotionally is often more helpful than correcting where they are factually.

Common time-related concerns and gentle responses:

When they worry about picking up children from school, "The children are safe and taken care of. Let's have some tea together."

If they insist it's time to cook dinner at breakfast, "Good thinking about dinner. Right now, let's enjoy this morning meal."

When they ask repeatedly what time it is: "We have plenty of time together. What would you like to do?"

These responses acknowledge their concerns without correcting their perception of time, reducing the anxiety that often accompanies temporal confusion.

Working with their timeline:

Sometimes, entering their timeframe temporarily can provide comfort. If they believe they're young and need to call their mother, you might say, "Your mother loves you very much" rather than explaining she died decades ago. This honors their emotional need for connection without causing the pain of re-experiencing loss.

The goal isn't deception - it's compassion.

When urgency strikes:

Time confusion often creates a sense of urgency about things that don't actually need immediate attention. Rather than explaining why they're wrong, try redirecting: "That sounds important. Let's sit down and talk about it," or "We'll take care of that together."

This approach maintains trust and reduces the agitation that comes from being constantly corrected, preparing you for the more hands-on aspects of caregiving we'll explore in Chapter 6, where this same patient, flexible mindset becomes essential.

When Memory Misplaces Everything Important:

When someone with dementia can't find something, they're often experiencing genuine distress that goes far beyond the inconvenience of a misplaced item. The confusion and frustration can quickly escalate into panic, especially when they believe the missing object is crucial to their safety or daily routine. Understanding this emotional layer helps you respond with the calm, supportive approach they need.

The item might be lost, misplaced, or simply forgotten entirely. Your role isn't to solve the mystery but to provide calm support and gentle assistance without making the person feel foolish or incapable.

This situation requires the same patient communication skills we discussed in Chapter 4, combined with the acceptance of confusion we explored earlier in this chapter. Fighting their distress or launching into detective mode often increases their anxiety rather than helping them feel secure.

Key principles for helping with lost items:

- Help look without making a big production of the search
- Offer alternatives if the original item can't be found
- Stay calm and matter-of-fact, avoiding phrases like "don't you remember?"

Robert was helping his neighbor when she became upset because she couldn't find her purse. Instead of launching into an extensive search or asking detailed questions about where she last saw it, Robert simply said, "Let's look together." His tone remained casual and reassuring, treating this as a normal, solvable situation.

They checked a few obvious places calmly and quietly. Robert didn't interrogate her about her movements or suggest places that might make her feel confused about her own actions. When they didn't find it immediately, he offered, "Would this small bag work for now?" pointing to a similar bag nearby.

She readily accepted it, and her distress disappeared.

Later, Robert quietly mentioned the missing purse to her daughter, who found it the next day in the refrigerator. But in that moment, solving the immediate emotional need was far more important than solving the practical mystery.

Common lost item scenarios:

Glasses often end up in unusual places - check the bathroom, kitchen counter, or even the freezer. Rather than questioning their placement logic, simply help look in likely spots while maintaining normal conversation.

Important documents may be "hidden" for safekeeping in places that made sense at the time but seem random now. Offer reassurance that paperwork can be handled later while focusing on their immediate concern.

Clothing items sometimes get put away in unexpected locations. If the specific piece can't be found, suggest similar alternatives without making them feel bad about the missing item.

Avoiding common mistakes:

Don't ask "Where did you put it?" or "When did you last see it?" These questions highlight their memory loss and can increase frustration. Instead, simply start looking together in reasonable places.

Avoid turning the search into a teaching moment about organization or memory strategies. Your goal is comfort, not improvement.

When items are genuinely lost:

Sometimes things are truly gone, donated, thrown away, or placed somewhere that defies logic. This reality doesn't diminish their distress or your role in providing comfort. Focus on meeting their emotional needs rather than recovering the physical object.

The patience and flexibility you develop handling these situations prepare you well for the personal care challenges we'll address in Chapter 6, where the same calm, supportive approach becomes even more crucial when helping with intimate daily tasks.

Steering Conversations Without Stirring Storms

Sometimes repetition and confusion create loops that feel stuck or distressing, both for the person with dementia and for you as their helper. When the same worried question surfaces for the tenth time, or when confusion about a situation seems to be building rather than settling, gentle redirection can provide relief for everyone involved.

The key is making the redirect feel natural and appealing, not like you're dismissing their concerns.

Redirection isn't about ignoring their needs or cutting them off - it's about offering their mind a different path when the current one leads to frustration. This technique builds directly on the communication strategies from Chapter 4, using your calm presence and gentle guidance to create a more peaceful experience.

Effective redirection strategies include:

· Offer an alternative activity that matches their current energy level

· Use transition phrases like "while we're thinking about that" or "speaking of..."

· Make the redirect about moving toward something pleasant, not away from something problematic

Marcus was spending an afternoon with his uncle when he became fixated on a confusing memory of his car keys, repeatedly asking where they were and becoming increasingly agitated. Each answer Marcus provided seemed to fuel more questions and worry rather than providing reassurance.

Instead of continuing to address the keys directly, Marcus said, "While we're thinking about that, would you like to see what's happening in the garden?" He guided his uncle to the window where they could see birds at the feeder. The change of scene and focus naturally shifted his attention away from the confusing loop.

The key anxiety dissolved within minutes.

Twenty minutes later, when his uncle mentioned the keys again, it was with much less distress, and Marcus was able to use the same gentle redirect. He learned that sometimes the kindest response to confusion is simply offering something else to focus on.

Natural transition techniques:

"Speaking of time, look how beautiful the light is coming through that window."

"That reminds me, would you like some tea?"

"While we're sitting here, tell me about this photograph."

These phrases acknowledge their concern without dismissing it, then smoothly guide attention toward something more manageable and pleasant.

Matching energy levels:

If they're agitated, offer calming activities like looking through photo albums or listening to familiar music. When they seem restless, suggest gentle movement, such as walking to another room or stepping outside for a brief walk.

The goal is meeting them where they are emotionally while providing a pathway to greater comfort.

When redirection doesn't work immediately:

Sometimes the first attempt doesn't take hold, and that's completely normal. Stay patient and try again with a different approach or activity. Your calm persistence often matters more than finding the perfect redirect on the first try.

Recap of Key Points

Repetition and confusion aren't problems to be solved - they're part of how dementia affects the brain. Your role as a helper is to respond with grace rather than correction. Remember that each repeated question feels fresh to them, and that time confusion is common and usually harmless. That gentle redirection works better than lengthy explanations. Most importantly, your calm, consistent responses provide the reassurance and safety they're truly seeking.

Action Steps

Practice responding to repeated questions with the same patient tone you'd use the first time. Develop gentle redirect phrases that feel natural to you. When confusion arises, focus on the emotion behind it rather than the facts within the questions.

While repetition and confusion can feel overwhelming at first, they're manageable with patience and the right approach. However, some helpers worry most about the more personal aspects of care - helping with daily tasks like eating, dressing, or personal hygiene. In Chapter 6, we'll explore how to handle personal care situations with dignity and confidence.

Personal Care Without Panic

When Caring Feels Too Personal

PERSONAL CARE REPRESENTS ONE of the most intimate aspects of dementia caregiving, and it's natural to feel uncertain about crossing these boundaries. The key lies in approaching these moments with the same respect and dignity you would want for yourself during vulnerable times.

Understanding the Emotional Layer

Personal care isn't just about physical tasks - it carries deep emotional weight for both you and the person receiving care. Many people with dementia feel embarrassed about needing help with basic tasks they've managed independently their entire adult lives. Your approach can either amplify these feelings or help minimize them through gentle, respectful support.

Dignity First: The Foundation of All Personal Care

Every interaction during personal care should prioritize the person's dignity above efficiency or convenience.

This means speaking before you act, preserving privacy whenever possible, and moving at their pace rather than rushing through tasks.

Daisy was helping her aunt get dressed for a doctor's appointment when she noticed her aunt had put her blouse on backwards. Her first instinct was to fix it quickly, but instead she paused and asked gently, "Would you like me to help adjust your blouse?" Her aunt looked down, noticed the issue, and nodded. Together, they slowly turned the blouse around, with Daisy providing just enough assistance to make it easier. Later, her aunt thanked her for "being so patient with an old lady."

The Basics: Bathroom, Clothing, and Hygiene Support

Personal care doesn't require medical training - it requires common sense, gentleness, and understanding that you're supporting basic human needs.

- Bathroom assistance: Offer help without assuming it's needed. "Would you like me to walk with you to the bathroom?" respects the person's autonomy while providing safety support

- Clothing guidance: Help them choose appropriate clothes while maintaining their independence. If something is worn incorrectly, ask if they'd like help rather than immediately correcting it

- Basic hygiene support: This might involve offering a warm washcloth for face and hands, helping with teeth brushing, or gently reminding about forgotten routines

George noticed his father-in-law had been wearing the same shirt for three days during his weekend visit. Instead of pointing this out directly, he laid out a fresh shirt on the bed and said, "I thought you might like a clean shirt for our trip to the garden center today." His father-in-law made the switch without embarrassment or resistance.

When to Step In: Reading the Signals

Learning the difference between when someone needs help and when they want help is crucial. Stepping in too quickly can feel invasive, while waiting too long might compromise safety.

Watch for subtle signs: someone who struggles with buttons for several minutes, looks confused about clothing choices, or seems uncomfortable with hygiene might need gentle offers of assistance. Always respect "no" when it's safe to do so - you can check back later or offer help differently.

Preserving Independence: Supporting Rather Than Taking Over

The goal isn't doing everything for someone - it's helping them do as much as possible for themselves while providing necessary support.

Use the "hand-over-hand" approach, placing your hands gently over theirs to guide familiar motions. Break tasks into smaller steps rather than overwhelming them with complex instructions. Celebrate small successes and acknowledge what they can do independently.

Handling Awkward Moments

Embarrassing situations will happen - clothing mishaps, bathroom accidents, or hygiene issues. Your response can either preserve dignity or create unnecessary shame.

Stay calm and matter-of-fact. Focus on solutions rather than problems. "Let's get you into some fresh clothes" works better than discussing accidents. Maintain privacy and avoid unnecessarily sharing these incidents.

Daisy found her uncle in soiled clothes, looking mortified. Instead of making a fuss, she simply said, "Let's get you cleaned up and into some comfortable clothes." She helped him to the bathroom, provided a warm washcloth, and laid out fresh clothing while maintaining gentle conversation about their day plans. Later, he thanked her for "not making me feel like a child."

Moving Forward

Personal care becomes easier with practice and patience. Your calm, respectful approach matters more than perfect technique. Remember that preserving dignity while ensuring safety and comfort is always the priority.

Eating, Routines, and Familiar Comforts

Soup, Stories, and Sunday Afternoons

FOOD REPRESENTS FAR MORE than nutrition for someone with dementia - it's connection, routine, and familiarity wrapped into something essential. Your role isn't to be a nutritionist or enforce perfect eating habits. It's to make mealtimes feel safe, unhurried, and pleasant.

Think about mealtime as an experience rather than a task. The goal shifts from getting someone to eat everything on the plate to creating moments of comfort and connection. When you sit down with someone who has dementia, you're offering presence alongside the meal.

Mealtime Magic: Creating Calm Around Food and Eating

Creating a peaceful eating environment starts before the food arrives. Just as we learned in Chapter 6 about approaching personal care with calm energy, your demeanor around meals sets the tone for the entire experience.

Simple strategies that make mealtimes easier:

· Focus on the atmosphere, not the amount consumed. A peaceful meal where someone eats half the sandwich is better than a stressful meal where they finish everything

· Offer choices between two simple options rather than asking open-ended questions. "Would you like tea or coffee?" works better than "What would you like to drink?"

· Sit with them if possible. Eating together, even if you're just having a cup of tea, makes the experience social rather than clinical

· Remove distractions like loud television or busy patterns on tablecloths that might confuse or overwhelm

Ian learned this lesson one afternoon while helping his father-in-law. He had prepared a full lunch - soup, sandwich, fruit, and cookies - and grew frustrated when his father-in-law only picked at the soup. "I thought I was failing," Ian later reflected. "But then he started telling me about the soup his mother used to make, and we spent an hour just talking. I realized the soup was just the starting point for something much more meaningful."

The conversation mattered more than the calories consumed.

Routine as Comfort

People with dementia often find security in familiar patterns. If someone always had coffee at three in the afternoon or preferred breakfast foods for dinner, these preferences become even more important as their world feels increasingly unpredictable.

Notice what brings comfort. Does someone light up when smelling cinnamon? Do they always reach for the same coffee cup? These small details aren't quirks to correct - they're anchors of familiarity in a confusing time.

Elizabeth discovered this while spending weekends with her neighbor. She noticed that her neighbor always wanted toast cut diagonally and became agitated when it was served differently. "At first I thought she was being picky," Elizabeth explained. "Then I realized this tiny thing made her feel like the world still made sense. Now I always cut her toast the same way, and she smiles every time."

When Eating Becomes Difficult

As dementia progresses, physical challenges with eating may emerge. Someone might forget how to use utensils, have trouble swallowing, or lose interest in food entirely. These changes connect to what we explored in previous chapters about accepting new realities without panic.

Your response matters more than your solutions. Staying calm when someone struggles helps them feel secure rather than embarrassed. If using a fork becomes confusing, offering finger foods isn't giving up - it's adapting with dignity.

Remember that mealtimes will eventually become more about presence than nutrition. The warmth you bring to these moments creates a comfort that nourishes in ways food alone cannot. This foundation of calm presence will become especially important as we explore emotional challenges in the next chapter.

Riding the Wave of Daily Rhythms

Routines provide structure and predictability in a world that can feel increasingly confusing. Rather than imposing your own schedule, learn to recognize and support the patterns that already exist. Even small routines - like having tea at 3 PM or watching a particular TV program - can anchor someone's day.

Think of yourself as joining an existing rhythm rather than creating a new one. Just as we learned in Chapter 6 about approaching personal care with calm awareness, understanding daily patterns requires observation and respect for what already works.

Before your visit, gather routine information:

· Ask the primary caregiver about established routines. When does this person usually eat? What time do they typically rest? What are their preferred activities?

· Don't rush transitions between activities. Allow extra time for transitions, and give gentle warnings: "In a few minutes, we'll have our afternoon tea."

· If a routine gets disrupted, don't panic. Flexibility matters more than perfect timing. The goal is comfort, not rigid adherence to a schedule

Diana discovered the importance of routine when she tried to surprise her aunt with an early dinner. "I thought I was being helpful by having everything ready at 4:30

instead of 5:30," she explained. "But she became agitated and kept asking what was wrong, why we were eating so early. Once I understood that 5:30 was her time, everything went much smoother. She needed that predictability."

Reading the Natural Flow

Every person with dementia has internal rhythms that persist even as cognitive abilities change. Some people feel most alert in the morning, while others come alive in the afternoon. Some need frequent small breaks, while others prefer longer periods of activity followed by extended rest.

Watch for these natural patterns during your time together. Does someone seem more talkative after lunch? Do they get restless around the same time each day? These observations help you work with their natural flow rather than against it.

The communication techniques from Chapter 4 become especially valuable here. Instead of asking "What do you want to do now?" try "It's almost time for your afternoon walk. Would you like to get your sweater?"

When Routines Feel Disrupted

Sometimes routines that once brought comfort become sources of confusion or distress. Someone might insist on getting dressed for work decades after retirement, or repeatedly prepare for an appointment that doesn't exist. These moments require the gentle redirection skills we've been building throughout previous chapters.

Edward faced this challenge when he visited his neighbor, who kept insisting that he pick up his children from school. His children were now adults with families of their own. "At first I tried to explain that his kids were grown up," Edward recalled. "But that just made him more upset. Then I learned to say, 'The kids are taken care of today. Let's have some coffee while we wait.' That usually helped him relax."

Creating Micro-Routines

Even during shorter visits, you can establish small patterns that provide comfort. Maybe you always start by sitting in the same chair and asking about their day. Perhaps you end each visit by looking through a photo album together. These mini-routines create familiarity within your time together.

The key is consistency without rigidity. If the usual routine isn't working on a particular day, adapt gracefully. Remember that the goal is to create a sense of safety and predictability, not to follow rules.

These routine-building skills become especially important when emotions run high - both theirs and yours. As we'll explore in the next chapter, maintaining familiar patterns can help prevent or ease emotional storms that sometimes arise in dementia care.

The Secret Lives of Comfort Objects

People with dementia often develop strong attachments to particular objects - a favorite sweater, a worn photograph, a coffee mug, or even something that might seem unusual to others. These items provide emotional security and a sense of identity. Your job is to respect and support these attachments, not question them.

Think of comfort objects as emotional anchors in a world that feels increasingly uncertain. Just as we learned in previous chapters about accepting rather than correcting, these attachments deserve the same gentle understanding we've practiced with communication and routines.

Guidelines for supporting comfort objects:

· Never remove or "correct" a comfort object unless it poses a genuine safety risk. If someone wants to carry around a purse all day or wear the same cardigan, that's perfectly fine

· If a comfort object gets lost or needs washing, have a gentle plan for temporary substitutes. Sometimes, a similar item can provide comfort while the original is unavailable

· Understand that the attachment isn't always logical, and that's okay. A wooden spoon might represent cooking and nurturing. A small pillow might provide the comfort of home

Steven was puzzled when his mother insisted on carrying a small toolbox with her everywhere during his visits. "I kept trying to put it away, thinking it was clutter," he admitted. "But then my sister explained that Dad had been a carpenter, and Mom had always helped him organize his tools. That toolbox wasn't random - it was her connection to fifty years of working alongside the person she loved most."

The Hidden Meaning in Everyday Items

What appears meaningless to you might hold deep significance for someone with dementia. A tissue box becomes a treasure chest. A magazine becomes a letter from a friend. A kitchen towel transforms into a soothing baby blanket.

These connections often relate to roles that once defined someone's identity. A woman who spent decades as a teacher might clutch notebooks and pencils. A man who worked in an office might carry around file folders. Rather than seeing these as confusion, recognize them as attempts to maintain connection with who they've always been.

Lisa learned this lesson while helping her neighbor, who insisted on "folding laundry" every afternoon using the same three towels. "At first I thought I should give her more towels to make it more productive," Lisa explained. "But I realized she wasn't trying to be productive - she was finding comfort in a familiar motion that had brought her satisfaction for decades."

Working With, Not Against

When someone becomes attached to an unusual comfort object, your response sets the tone for the entire interaction. The calm presence we've practiced in personal care situations applies perfectly here. Getting frustrated or trying to logic away the attachment creates distress for everyone involved.

Instead, become curious about the object's significance. Ask gentle questions. "That's a beautiful scarf you're holding. Does it remind you of something special?" Sometimes the person can share the connection. Other times, the meaning remains private, and that's perfectly acceptable.

Practical Considerations

Sometimes comfort objects create minor challenges. Someone might refuse to let go of an item during meals or personal care. The solutions usually involve gentle negotiation rather than forceful removal.

Try saying, "Let's put your special book right here on the table where you can see it while we eat lunch." Or "Would you like to hold this while I help with your sweater, then we'll put it right back?"

These small accommodations honor the emotional importance while allowing necessary activities to continue. Remember that these objects often become more significant as other abilities decline. What seems like a simple attachment today might become a crucial source of comfort tomorrow - knowledge that will serve us well as we explore the emotional challenges in our next chapter.

Gentle Joys for Overwhelmed Minds

The best activities for someone with dementia are often the simplest ones. You don't need elaborate entertainment or complex projects. Look for activities that gently engage the senses, connect to familiar experiences, and allow for success regardless of cognitive changes.

Think of activities as opportunities for connection rather than tasks to complete. Just as we've learned in previous chapters about following someone's lead in communication and personal care, the same principle applies to shared activities.

Guidelines for choosing meaningful activities:

· Choose activities with no "wrong" way to do them. Folding towels, looking through photo albums, listening to familiar music, or sorting buttons can be soothing and engaging

· Follow their lead and energy level. If they seem tired, choose quieter activities. If they're restless, gentle movement or simple tasks might help

· Remember that the activity itself isn't the goal - connection and comfort are. If you spend an hour just sitting together watching birds outside the window, that's a perfectly valuable way to spend time

Sarah learned about simple pleasures when she brought a bag of colorful fabric scraps to sort with her grandmother. "I thought we might make something with them," she said. "But Grandma was perfectly happy just feeling the different textures and telling me about dresses she used to sew. We never made anything, but she smiled the whole time and seemed so peaceful. I realized I had been overthinking what would make her happy."

Activities That Connect to Memory

The most engaging activities often tap into skills and interests that remain familiar even as other abilities change. Someone who once loved cooking might enjoy stirring ingredients or kneading dough. A former gardener might find comfort in touching soil or watering plants, even indoors.

These connections don't require perfect memory or execution. The comfort comes from familiar motions and sensations rather than achieving specific outcomes.

When David brought his father newspapers to read, his father couldn't follow the stories anymore, but still enjoyed the ritual of turning pages and the feel of newsprint between his fingers.

Sensory Comfort

Simple sensory experiences often provide deep satisfaction. Soft textures, pleasant scents, familiar sounds, or gentle visual stimulation can create moments of peace and engagement. A basket of smooth stones to handle, lavender sachets to smell, or old photographs to examine can occupy attention in soothing ways.

Music deserves special mention here. Songs from someone's youth often remain accessible long after other memories fade. Don't worry about having the perfect playlist - even humming familiar tunes together can create a connection.

Following Natural Rhythms

Pay attention to natural energy patterns throughout your visit. Some people feel most social in the morning, while others come alive later in the day. Some need frequent gentle activity, while others prefer longer periods of quiet companionship.

The routine awareness we discussed earlier in this chapter applies to activities as well. If someone always enjoys afternoon walks, suggest a gentle stroll. If they were night owls, don't force morning activities during later visits.

The Thread That Connects

What connects all these elements - eating, routines, comfort objects, and simple pleasures - is respect for individual preferences and history. What comforts one person might not comfort another. Your role is to observe, support, and adapt rather than direct or change.

The calm presence you've been practicing throughout previous chapters becomes your greatest tool here. When you approach activities without pressure or expectations, you create space for genuine moments of joy and connection.

While routines and familiar comforts provide stability, there will be moments when emotions rise - both theirs and yours. Understanding how to navigate these emotional moments with grace and confidence is what we'll explore next, giving you the tools to stay calm even when feelings run high.

When Emotions Rise - Theirs and Yours

When Dementia Amplifies Every Emotion

Emotions don't disappear with dementia - they often become more intense and immediate. When the brain's usual filters and coping mechanisms are affected, feelings can surge without warning, like sudden weather changes. What might once have been mild frustration can become overwhelming distress, or a small worry can feel catastrophic.

The emotional centers of the brain often remain active even when other functions decline, which means your loved one can feel deeply even when they can't express those feelings clearly. Understanding this helps you respond with compassion rather than confusion when emotions seem to come from nowhere.

Key points about heightened emotions:

· Emotions may feel more raw because the brain struggles to process and regulate them as it once did

· Feelings can shift quickly from calm to upset without obvious triggers that make sense to you

· Past emotions and memories may surface unexpectedly, creating confusion about time and place

· Physical discomfort, hunger, or fatigue can significantly amplify emotional responses

Brooklyn was helping her aunt one afternoon when her aunt suddenly became tearful, insisting that she needed to pick up her children from school. Her children were grown adults with families of their own, but in that moment, her aunt's worry felt completely real and urgent. Brooklyn learned that arguing with the logic wouldn't help - acknowledging the feeling behind the concern was what mattered.

"You're such a caring mother," she said gently. "Your children are safe."

The tears gradually subsided as her aunt felt heard rather than corrected.

Your Emotions Matter Too

Caregiving stirs up complex feelings in helpers as well. You might feel sad watching someone you love struggle, frustrated when communication breaks down, or guilty when you need a break. These feelings are completely normal and deserve attention.

Remember the communication techniques we discussed in Chapter 4 - they become especially important during emotional moments. When someone with dementia is upset, your calm presence often matters more than finding the perfect words.

Common emotional challenges for helpers:

· Grief over watching personality changes in someone you love

· Frustration when repeated explanations don't seem to help

· Anxiety about making mistakes or saying the wrong thing

· Exhaustion from emotional ups and downs throughout a single visit

Logan discovered this when his grandfather became agitated during their weekly visit, repeatedly asking for his wife, who had passed away years earlier. Initially, Logan felt overwhelmed and sad, unsure whether to remind his grandfather about the loss or play along. He learned that neither approach was always right - instead, he focused on the emotion behind the question.

"You miss her so much," Logan would say, which usually brought comfort without requiring difficult explanations.

Strategies That Actually Work

Building on the routine-centered approach from Chapter 7, emotional regulation often improves when basic needs are met. Before addressing big feelings, check if your loved one is hungry, tired, too hot, or uncomfortable.

Simple emotional support techniques:

· Validate feelings even when the situation seems confusing

- Use a gentle touch if it's welcomed and appropriate
- Speak slowly and softly during emotional moments
- Avoid taking emotional outbursts personally
- Give yourself permission to step away briefly if needed

The goal isn't to fix every emotional moment but to provide a steady, caring presence. As we'll explore in Chapter 9, some behaviors and emotional responses follow patterns, especially during certain times of day, which can help you prepare and respond more effectively.

Your emotional well-being directly impacts your ability to help others.

Take care of yourself, too.

Keep Your Cool When Chaos Strikes

Your emotional state becomes an anchor in stormy moments. When someone with dementia is upset, they often mirror the energy around them. If you remain calm and steady, it creates a stabilizing presence that can help de-escalate the situation. This doesn't mean suppressing your own feelings, but rather managing them so they don't add to the emotional intensity.

The communication principles from Chapter 4 become even more critical when emotions run high. Your tone of voice, body language, and facial expressions communicate as much as your words - sometimes more.

Essential strategies for staying calm:

· Take slow, deep breaths to keep your own nervous system calm

· Lower your voice and slow your movements when emotions are high

· Remember that their emotional storm isn't about you - it's about their experience of confusion or distress

· Use the familiar comfort techniques from Chapter 7 to help restore stability

Edward was visiting his father when his father became agitated, accusing Edward of stealing his wallet. Edward's first instinct was to defend himself and search frantically for the wallet to prove his innocence. Instead, he took a moment to breathe and said, "That must be really worrying. Let's look for it together." His calm response helped his father feel supported rather than defensive, and they found the wallet in his father's jacket pocket.

The accusation was forgotten, but the feeling of being helped was remembered.

When You Feel Overwhelmed

Sometimes, keeping your cool feels impossible, especially when emotions escalate quickly or accusations feel personal. Recognizing your own emotional triggers helps you respond more thoughtfully rather than react impulsively.

Building on the repetition-handling skills from Chapter 5, remember that emotional outbursts often follow similar patterns. What looks like random chaos usually has underlying causes - physical discomfort, confusion about time or place, or unmet needs.

Warning signs you need a moment:

- Your heart rate increases significantly
- You feel the urge to argue or correct aggressively
- Your voice starts to rise or become sharp
- You feel personally attacked by their words or actions

It's completely acceptable to say, "I'm going to get you some water," and step away for thirty seconds to collect yourself. This brief pause can prevent situations from escalating and gives both of you a chance to reset.

Susan learned this lesson when her mother repeatedly insisted that strangers were living in her house. Initially, Susan would launch into detailed explanations about how those "strangers" were actually family members. These conversations always ended with both of them frustrated and upset. Susan discovered that acknowledging the feeling worked better: "That would be scary to have people you don't recognize in your home. You're safe here with me."

Practical De-escalation Techniques

Remember the routine-based approach from Chapter 7 - emotional regulation often improves when you address basic needs first. Before diving into complex emotional discussions, check whether hunger, fatigue, or discomfort might be contributing to the distress.

Quick de-escalation steps:

- Validate their emotions without agreeing with the confused details

- Offer simple physical comfort, like a gentle hand on their shoulder

- Redirect to calming activities they've enjoyed before

- Use their name frequently to help ground them in the present

- Suggest familiar foods or drinks as a comfort measure

These techniques prepare you for the more challenging behaviors we'll explore in Chapter 9, where timing and environmental factors play crucial roles in managing difficult moments. Understanding your own emotional responses gives you the foundation to handle even more complex situations with confidence.

Your calmness becomes their anchor.

Practice these techniques when emotions are low so they're ready when storms arise.

Turning Heat into Harmony

De-escalation isn't about fixing the problem or changing someone's mind - it's about reducing the emotional temperature in the room. Simple techniques can make a significant difference in helping someone feel safer and more settled. The goal is to move from chaos toward calm, not to solve whatever triggered the upset.

Building on the communication strategies from Chapter 4, your approach during heated moments can either fuel the fire or help it settle naturally. Remember that the brain changes in dementia make it harder for someone to calm themselves down once they're upset, so your steady presence becomes their pathway back to peace.

Core de-escalation principles:

- Validate their feelings without necessarily agreeing with their interpretation of events
- Use gentle distraction by suggesting a simple, comforting activity
- Give them physical and emotional space while staying nearby and available
- Keep your voice soft and your movements slow and predictable

Eleanor was caring for her neighbor when he became increasingly frustrated trying to button his shirt. The more he struggled, the more upset he became. Instead of taking over or offering detailed instructions, Eleanor sat down nearby and said, "Those buttons can be tricky. Would you like some tea while you work on that?" The simple offer of tea shifted his attention just enough to break the cycle of frustration, and he was able to complete the task at his own pace.

The Power of Simple Redirections

Just like the familiar routines we discussed in Chapter 7 provide comfort and stability, familiar activities can serve as emotional anchors during difficult moments. The key is offering something appealing without making it feel like you're dismissing their current concerns.

Effective redirection techniques:

- Suggest looking at photo albums together
- Offer a favorite snack or beverage
- Mention a person they enjoy talking about
- Propose a gentle activity like folding laundry or sorting items
- Ask for their help with something simple

Charles discovered this approach when his grandmother became agitated about nonexistent missed appointments. Rather than explaining the confusion, he said, "You're always so organized with appointments. Could you help me organize these papers?" Her desire to be helpful redirected her focus, and the anxiety about the appointments faded away naturally.

When Nothing Seems to Work

Sometimes emotions run so high that standard techniques don't immediately help. Drawing from the repetition-handling skills in Chapter 5, remember that persistence and patience often matter more than perfect technique. What doesn't work in one moment might work perfectly five minutes later.

Signs it's time to try a different approach:

- Their distress continues to escalate despite your efforts
- You feel your own frustration rising significantly

· The current environment feels too stimulating or chaotic

· Physical needs like hunger or fatigue might be contributing factors

During these moments, the emotional regulation strategies from earlier in this chapter become essential. Take care of your own emotional state first, then return to helping them find calm.

Consider suggesting a change of scenery - moving to a different room, stepping outside briefly, or even just sitting in a different chair can sometimes break the cycle of distress. The familiar comfort strategies from Chapter 7 work especially well here: offering a soft blanket, playing gentle music, or providing a warm drink.

As we'll explore in Chapter 9, some challenging behaviors follow predictable patterns, especially related to time of day and environmental factors. Understanding these patterns helps you anticipate and prepare for difficult moments before they escalate.

The goal isn't perfection in every interaction.

Small improvements in emotional temperature make meaningful differences for everyone involved.

Holding Space Through Life's Hardest Moments

People with dementia often experience waves of grief as they sense something is different or missing, even if they can't articulate what it is. This sadness is real and valid, whether it's about recent losses or older grief that surfaces unexpectedly. Your role isn't to cheer them up or explain away their feelings, but to sit with them in their sadness and offer gentle comfort.

The communication techniques from Chapter 4 become especially important during these vulnerable moments. Your presence communicates care more powerfully than any words you might offer. Sometimes the most healing thing you can do is simply witness their pain without trying to fix it.

Essential approaches for holding emotional space:

- Allow tears and sadness without rushing to fix or change the mood
- Offer simple comfort like a tissue, a gentle touch, or a quiet presence
- Avoid phrases like "don't cry" or "everything's fine" - instead, try "I'm here with you."
- Let them express feelings, even if the details don't match your understanding of reality

Marcus was spending the afternoon with his grandmother when she suddenly began crying, saying she missed her mother. His grandmother's mother had passed away decades earlier, but the grief felt fresh and immediate. Rather than reminding her of the timeline, Marcus simply said, "She sounds like she was very special to you. Tell me about her." They spent the next hour looking through old photos, and his grandmother's tears gradually gave way to warm memories and gentle smiles.

When Grief Feels Overwhelming

Drawing from the emotional regulation strategies discussed earlier in this chapter, remember that intense grief episodes often pass more quickly when they're acknowledged rather than redirected. As with the repetition-handling approach in Chapter 5, sometimes the best response is patient acceptance rather than active intervention.

Signs someone needs emotional space:

- They become withdrawn or unusually quiet
- Tears come without obvious triggers
- They mention people or places from long ago with fresh sadness
- They express feeling lost or confused about their life situation

Building on the familiar comfort techniques from Chapter 7, simple physical comforts can provide grounding during emotional storms. A warm blanket, a cup of tea, or familiar music can offer stability when feelings feel overwhelming.

Sarah learned this when her father became deeply sad during their visit, repeatedly saying he wanted to "go home" despite being in his own house for twenty years. She realized he wasn't talking about the physical building but about feeling at home in his own life. Instead of explaining where he was, she focused on creating a sense of emotional comfort. She made his favorite coffee and put on music from his younger years. She sat quietly beside him until the sadness lifted naturally.

Supporting Without Fixing

Remember the principles from Chapter 3 about letting go of trying to do everything perfectly. You cannot take away someone's grief or confusion, and trying to do so often increases their distress. Your job is to offer a steady, caring presence while they navigate difficult emotions.

Practical ways to provide support:

· Validate their feelings with simple statements like "that sounds really hard."

· Share the quiet without feeling pressure to fill it with conversation

· Offer gentle distractions only after acknowledging their emotions first

· Trust that difficult moments will pass, even if you can't control when

These skills prepare you for the more complex behavioral challenges we'll explore in Chapter 9, where timing patterns and environmental factors create additional layers of difficulty. Understanding how to hold emotional space gives you the confidence to handle whatever comes next.

Grief shared is grief lightened.

Your patient presence matters more than perfect words.

When Your Heart Hits the Wall

Caring for someone during emotional moments can be draining, and it's important to recognize when you've reached your limit. This isn't failure - it's self-awareness. Sometimes the kindest thing you can do is step back, regroup, or ask for help. Pushing through when you're emotionally depleted often makes situations worse for everyone involved.

Drawing on the communication principles from Chapter 4, remember that your emotional state directly affects the person you're helping. When you're overwhelmed, stressed, or frustrated, these feelings can amplify the dementia patient's distress rather than calm it.

Warning signs you need support:

- Notice physical signs of stress in your own body - tension, rapid heartbeat, or shallow breathing
- You feel angry or resentful during interactions
- Simple tasks feel impossibly difficult
- You're fighting back tears or feeling emotionally raw

It's okay to take a brief break in another room to collect yourself. Don't hesitate to call the primary caregiver if you feel out of your depth. Remember the lesson from Chapter 3 about letting go of perfectionism - recognizing your limits shows wisdom, not weakness.

Helen had been helping her uncle for several hours when he became increasingly agitated about wanting to go home, even though he was already in his own house. Nothing she tried seemed to help, and she could feel her own anxiety rising. She recognized that her stress was probably making things worse, so she called her cousin to come over early. "I think he might benefit from seeing a familiar face," she explained. Her cousin arrived within twenty minutes, and her uncle's agitation settled almost immediately.

Helen learned that knowing when to ask for help was just as important as knowing how to provide it.

Emotional Recovery Strategies

Building on the familiar comfort techniques from Chapter 7, you need your own comfort strategies for emotional recovery. Just as routines provide stability for people with dementia, having personal practices for managing stress helps you stay resilient.

Quick emotional reset techniques:

· Step outside for fresh air and a few deep breaths

· Splash cool water on your face or wrists

· Call a friend who understands your situation

· Listen to calming music for a few minutes

· Practice the grounding techniques that work best for you

Remember the repetition-handling skills from Chapter 5 - difficult moments often repeat, but so do your opportunities to respond with patience and care. Each challenging interaction teaches you something valuable for next time.

Building Your Support Network

The emotional regulation strategies discussed throughout this chapter work best when you have backup support. Like the teamwork approach emphasized in Chapter 2, caring for someone with dementia should never be a solo endeavor, even during short visits.

Essential support elements:

- Have contact numbers readily available for the primary caregiver
- Know which neighbors or friends can step in if needed
- Understand basic emergency procedures and contact information
- Identify your own emotional support people for debriefing after difficult visits

Thomas discovered the importance of support networks when his grandmother became inconsolable during what was supposed to be a pleasant afternoon visit. He felt completely helpless watching her cry without being able to comfort her. After calling her daughter for guidance, he learned that these episodes were becoming more common and that the best approach was simply to sit quietly with her until they passed.

The experience taught him that asking for guidance wasn't admitting defeat - it was ensuring better care for his grandmother.

Moving Forward with Confidence

Emotional moments in dementia care can feel intense and unpredictable. Still, the skills you've learned in this chapter provide a solid foundation. Understanding that emotions can amplify, knowing how to de-escalate situations, holding space for grief, and recognizing your own limits give you the tools to handle whatever arises.

As we move into Chapter 9, we'll explore how certain behaviors follow predictable patterns related to time of day and environmental factors, building on everything you've learned about emotional regulation and communication.

Sundowning and Challenging Behaviors

When Afternoon Energy Hits Empty

IT WAS FOUR O'CLOCK on a Tuesday afternoon when Samantha called her daughter in a panic. "Something's wrong with your father," she whispered into the phone. "He's been fine all day, but now he's pacing around asking for his mother and saying he needs to go home. We've been in this house for thirty years." What Samantha was witnessing wasn't unusual - it was sundowning, a pattern where confusion, restlessness, and agitation increase as daylight fades.

Late afternoon and early evening can bring unexpected challenges for people with dementia. This isn't about stubbornness or being difficult - it's often a combination of fatigue, changing light, and disrupted internal clocks that can make this time of day particularly unsettling.

Common sundowning triggers include:

- Shadows and changing light that create visual confusion

- Mental fatigue that builds throughout the day
- Disrupted internal body clocks
- Hunger or thirst that hasn't been addressed
- Overstimulation from the day's activities

Thomas had been having pleasant conversations with his son all afternoon. As evening approached, he became convinced that strangers were in his house. His son learned that closing curtains early and turning on familiar lamps helped reduce the shadowy confusion that seemed to trigger his father's distress. The key wasn't arguing about who the "strangers" were - it was creating an environment that felt safer and more familiar.

Understanding what might be driving the behavior helps you respond with compassion rather than frustration. When someone with dementia becomes agitated in the evening, that person is often experiencing genuine distress - even if the cause isn't immediately clear to you.

Practical strategies for sundowning:

Create consistent evening routines. Start winding down activities an hour before the usual sundowning time. This might mean switching from active conversations to quieter activities, such as looking through photo albums or listening to gentle music.

Manage lighting carefully. Close curtains or blinds before shadows become prominent, and turn on warm, familiar lighting throughout the space. Avoid harsh overhead lights that can create confusing shadows.

Address basic needs early. Make sure the person has had enough to eat and drink before late afternoon arrives. Sometimes what looks like behavioral changes is actually hunger or discomfort.

Stay calm yourself. Remember the emotional regulation techniques from Chapter 8 - your calm presence can help steady someone who's feeling confused or frightened. Your anxiety will only add to theirs.

When challenging behaviors emerge, resist the urge to correct or argue with the person's reality. Samantha learned this when her husband started insisting he needed to pick up the children from their sports activities - children who had been adults for decades, with their own transport. Instead of explaining that the children were grown, she began saying, "The children are safe and taken care of." This acknowledged his concern without creating conflict.

Redirecting rather than correcting often works better:

- "You're worried about them - that shows what a caring father you are."
- "Let's sit down together while we wait for news."
- "I can see this is important to you."

Sometimes the behavior isn't about the specific thing the person is saying - it's about an underlying feeling of worry, loneliness, or confusion. Addressing the feeling often helps more than addressing the words.

As we move into the next chapter on early-stage support, remember that sundowning and challenging behaviors can occur at any stage of dementia, but understanding these patterns helps you provide better support throughout the journey.

When Anxiety Takes the Wheel

When Florence started wringing her hands and repeating "I need to go, I need to go" over and over, her neighbor wasn't sure whether to try to calm her down or call someone for help. The repetitive movement and urgent tone felt alarming. Florence wasn't in immediate danger - she was experiencing the kind of restless agitation that can emerge when internal anxiety has nowhere to go.

Restlessness often stems from feelings that can't be easily expressed - discomfort, confusion, or a vague sense that something isn't right. Rather than trying to eliminate these feelings, your role is to provide a calm, steady presence that doesn't add to the existing anxiety.

Common triggers for restless behaviors:

- Physical discomfort that can't be clearly communicated
- Overstimulation from noise, lights, or too much activity
- Fatigue that makes processing information more difficult
- Changes in routine or environment that feel unsettling
- Medication side effects or timing issues

Isaiah found that when his wife became agitated in the evenings, sitting beside her and gently humming old songs she knew helped more than any words. Sometimes she would join in humming, and sometimes she would just gradually slow her restless movements. He learned that his calm presence was more powerful than any explanation he could offer about why she was feeling unsettled.

Practical responses to anxiety and agitation:

Don't take it personally. When someone with dementia becomes agitated, it's rarely about you or something you did wrong. The dementia patient's brain is struggling to process information or manage emotions, and you happened to be present when that struggle became visible.

Lower your own energy first. Remember the emotional regulation techniques from Chapter 8 - you can't help someone calm down if you're feeling anxious yourself. Take a deep breath, slow your movements, and soften your voice before you try to help.

Offer simple, repetitive activities. Folding washcloths, sorting through a box of familiar objects, or even just holding something soft can give restless hands something to do. The key is choosing activities that feel purposeful without being complicated.

Create physical comfort. Sometimes agitation comes from being too warm or too cold, or from sitting in an uncomfortable position. Check for simple physical needs before assuming the distress is purely emotional.

Use your voice as a tool. Speak more slowly and quietly than feels natural to you. Your calm tone can help regulate the person's emotional state, even when your words don't seem to be getting through.

When Florence started pacing and saying she needed to find her mother, her daughter's first instinct was to remind her that her mother had passed away years ago. But this only increased Florence's distress. Instead, her daughter learned to say, "Tell me about your mother," which allowed Florence to share memories and feel heard rather than corrected.

Validation often works better than correction:

- "You're thinking about her - she must have been special to you."
- "It sounds like you miss her."
- "She was lucky to have someone who cares so much."

Sometimes, challenging behaviors emerge when basic needs aren't met. Even so, they're just part of how the brain processes stress when dementia is present.

The goal isn't to eliminate all anxiety or agitation - that's not realistic. The goal is to provide steady, calm support that doesn't make the situation worse.

As we move into the next chapter on early-stage support, remember that the techniques you're learning for managing challenging behaviors will serve you throughout the dementia journey, adapting to different needs at different stages.

Protecting Without Pushing Back

The front door had been opened and closed six times in the past hour. Margaret kept putting on her coat, walking to the door, then taking the coat off again. Her daughter-in-law watched nervously, unsure whether to lock the door or let her go outside. The impulse to move, to go somewhere, felt urgent to Margaret, even though she couldn't articulate where she needed to be.

Wandering impulses often come from deep feelings - the need to find something familiar, to fulfill a responsibility that feels important, or simply to move when sitting still feels impossible. Fighting these impulses directly often increases distress, but you can redirect the energy in safer ways.

Understanding the "why" behind wandering:

- Need to find something or someone important
- Restlessness that has no clear outlet
- Following old routines that feel necessary
- Physical discomfort that movement might relieve
- Searching for a place that feels like "home."

Richard discovered that when his father felt the need to "go to work," taking a walk around the block together satisfied the impulse to move and be purposeful. By the time they returned home, the urgent feeling had often passed, and his father would settle into his chair without the same restlessness. The walk became a solution that honored the feeling without creating a battle.

Practical approaches to wandering behaviors:

Acknowledge the feeling behind the movement. Say "You seem like you need to go somewhere" rather than "You can't go out." This validates their experience without immediately creating conflict.

Offer safe alternatives for the movement impulse. Walking around the house, going to the garden, or even walking to the mailbox together can satisfy the need to move while keeping everyone safe.

Create gentle obstacles rather than firm barriers. Shoes that are harder to find, doors that require two steps to open, or simply walking alongside rather than blocking the path can slow down impulsive departures without creating confrontation.

Use distraction timing wisely. When someone is in the middle of a strong wandering impulse, distraction often doesn't work. But if you can catch the restlessness before it becomes urgent, offering an activity or snack might redirect the energy.

When Patricia started looking for her children every afternoon around three o'clock - the time she used to pick them up from school decades ago - her son learned to work with the pattern instead of against it. At 2:45, he would suggest they "go check on things" and take her for a drive around the neighborhood. This satisfied her need to be responsible for her children while keeping everyone safe.

Safety strategies that don't feel restrictive:

- ID bracelets or cards with contact information
- Door alarms that alert you without preventing exit
- Familiar photos or objects near exits that might prompt a pause
- Walking paths in yards or safe outdoor spaces

Remember the emotional regulation techniques from Chapter 8 - your own anxiety about safety can actually increase their restlessness. When you're calm and confident, it's easier to find creative solutions that work for everyone.

Sometimes wandering isn't about going somewhere specific - it's about the feeling of movement and purpose. Folding laundry, organizing a junk drawer, or even just walking back and forth in a long hallway can provide the physical activity and sense of accomplishment that satisfies the underlying need.

The goal isn't to eliminate all wandering impulses, but to channel them in directions that feel satisfying while maintaining safety.

As we transition to exploring early-stage support in the next chapter, remember that these redirection techniques work at every stage of dementia. However, the specific strategies may need to be adapted as needs change.

When Everything Falls Apart Anyway

It was one of those evenings where everything Dorothy tried seemed to make things worse. Her mother had been increasingly agitated since late afternoon, and nothing - not music, not tea, not familiar photos - seemed to help. Dorothy felt like she was failing, watching her mother pace and mutter, with an expression of deep distress that seemed to touch nothing.

Some days are simply harder than others, and that doesn't reflect on your caregiving abilities. Just as we all have days when we feel unsettled or uncomfortable without clear reasons, people with dementia can have periods when no amount of comfort or familiarity feels like enough.

Understanding difficult days:

· Dementia can create internal discomfort that has no clear solution

· Weather, medication changes, or physical factors you can't see might contribute

· Sometimes the brain is just having a harder time processing the world

· Your job isn't to fix every difficult moment - it's to stay calm and present through them

Michael learned to recognize when his wife was having what he called "a gray day" - times when her usual comforts didn't work and everything felt harder for both of them. Instead of trying harder to cheer her up, he learned to sit quietly nearby, offering gentle reassurance without pressure. He discovered that his calm acceptance of her difficult feelings often helped more than his attempts to change them.

<u>What to do when nothing seems to work</u>:

Lower your expectations for the moment. Instead of trying to create happiness or engagement, focus on preventing the situation from getting worse. Sometimes that's the best you can do, and it's enough.

Stay physically present without demanding interaction. Sit in the same room, move slowly, speak softly if you speak at all. Your calm energy can provide comfort even when nothing else seems to help.

Don't take it personally. When someone with dementia has a difficult day, it's not because you're doing something wrong or because they're rejecting your help. Their brain is struggling with something you can't see or fix.

Remember that difficult periods usually pass. Even when it doesn't feel like they will in the moment, most challenging episodes do end. Your job is to weather them together, not to make them disappear instantly.

Sometimes the most helpful thing you can do is simply not make the situation worse by adding your own anxiety to the mix. When Lisa's father became agitated, and nothing she tried helped, she learned to tell herself, "This is hard for both of us right now, and that's okay." This simple acceptance helped her stay calmer, which in turn helped him feel less overwhelmed.

Key reminders for challenging days:

- You can't control dementia, but you can control your response to it

- Comfort isn't always about making someone happy - sometimes it's about staying steady through difficulty

- The emotional regulation techniques from Chapter 8 matter most when things feel hardest

- Every challenging moment teaches you something about what might help next time

Looking ahead to different stages:

The specific challenges you face - sundowning, restlessness, difficult days - can look different depending on where someone is in their dementia journey. Early-stage dementia might lead to frustration over memory lapses. At the same time, later stages might involve greater physical restlessness or confusion about familiar people.

Understanding these patterns can help you adjust your approach and expectations as needs change over time.

While challenging behaviors can feel overwhelming in the moment, they're just one part of the caregiving experience. In our next chapter, we'll explore how your approach might shift depending on where someone is in their dementia journey - because what helps in early stages may look quite different from what brings comfort later on.

Early-Stage Support - Maintaining Connection

Spotting the First Warning Signs

EARLY-STAGE DEMENTIA OFTEN LOOKS like ordinary forgetfulness or stress, making it easy to miss or dismiss the significance of small changes. Understanding what you're actually seeing helps you offer the right kind of support without overstepping or underestimating someone's capabilities.

The challenge with recognizing early signs lies in their subtlety. Unlike the more obvious changes we discussed in the previous chapter regarding sundowning behaviors, early-stage symptoms blend into normal life variations. Most people have days when they forget where they put their keys or struggle to find the right word during a conversation.

The difference comes down to patterns and persistence.

What Early Changes Actually Look Like

Memory patterns that signal concern:

· Forgetting recent conversations or appointments while remembering distant events clearly

· Repeating questions or stories within the same conversation

· Missing important dates or events they've always remembered

· Difficulty learning new information or routines

Communication changes that stand out:

· Difficulty finding words or following complex conversations, especially in noisy environments

· Withdrawing from social situations they previously enjoyed

· Changes in writing or speaking patterns

· Trouble following multi-step instructions

Judgment and decision-making shifts:

· Changes in judgment or decision-making that seem out of character but are not obviously concerning

· Difficulty managing finances or making poor financial choices

· Problems with familiar tasks like cooking or driving routes they know well

· Confusion about time, place, or familiar faces

Lauren had always been the family organizer, the one who remembered everyone's birthdays and kept track of social events. When she started asking the same questions twice in a single phone call, her daughter initially attributed it to her being busy. It wasn't until Lauren missed two doctor's appointments in one month - something she'd never done in forty years - that the family realized something more significant was happening.

The key wasn't the individual incidents, but the pattern of changes in abilities that had always been her strengths.

Supporting Without Taking Over

When you notice these early signs in someone you care about, your instinct might be to jump in and start managing things for them. This approach often backfires, creating resistance and damaging the very relationship you're trying to protect.

Instead, focus on gentle support that preserves dignity:

Offer specific help rather than general assistance. Instead of saying "Do you need help with everything?" try "Would you like me to write down the appointment time while we're talking?"

Create subtle backup systems. If someone struggles with appointments, offer to put them in your calendar too, "so you can remind each other." This removes shame while providing practical support.

Stay connected to their world. People in early stages often feel isolated as they begin to notice their own changes. Regular check-ins, shared activities, and normal conversation help combat this isolation.

The communication strategies we covered in Chapter 4 become especially important during this stage. People experiencing early cognitive changes often feel frustrated and embarrassed by their difficulties. Your calm, patient presence provides reassurance that relationships can continue even as abilities change.

Remember that early-stage support isn't about fixing problems - it's about maintaining connection and providing gentle assistance that allows someone to function with dignity. As we'll explore in the next chapter about mid-stage changes, the nature of your support will evolve, but the foundation of respect and connection remains constant throughout every stage of this journey.

The goal is to help without unnecessarily taking away independence.

Helping Hands Without Taking Over

The goal in early-stage support is to help someone maintain their sense of competence and control while quietly filling in gaps where needed. This requires a delicate balance between offering assistance and allowing independence, always erring on the side of preserving dignity.

Unlike the more direct interventions we discussed for managing sundowning behaviors in Chapter 9, early-stage support operates through subtlety and partnership. The person you're helping still recognizes their own capabilities and wants to maintain control over their life decisions.

This makes your approach critical.

The Art of Invisible Assistance

Offering help as a partnership rather than taking over transforms potentially embarrassing situations into collaborative moments. Instead of saying "Let me handle your bills," try "Would you like me to help organize these papers with you?" The difference matters enormously to someone who's beginning to notice their own struggles.

Supporting decision-making rather than making decisions for them preserves autonomy while providing necessary backup. When Hope started having trouble following her doctor's complex medication schedule, her daughter didn't take over the pills completely. Instead, she sat with her mother during medication sorting, asking questions like "What did Dr. Smith say about the timing for this one?" This kept Hope in the decision-making role while ensuring important details weren't missed.

Acknowledging their expertise and experience while gently assisting with execution honors their lifetime of knowledge. Howard had been managing his finances for 50 years, but bank statements were starting to confuse him. Rather than taking over his accounts, his son asked Howard to teach him the system he'd always used, then offered to help with the calculations "to make sure we both understand the numbers the same way."

Practical Partnership Strategies

Create natural moments for collaboration:

- "I'm going to the grocery store anyway - want to ride along and help me remember what I need?"

· "I'm organizing my own paperwork today - would it help if we did yours at the same time?"

· "Let's both check our calendars and see what's coming up this week."

Use your presence as the intervention: Sometimes the help isn't in doing tasks differently, but in doing them together. The person feels more confident and makes fewer errors when tackling complex tasks with others.

Build in gentle double-checking: "Did I understand correctly that your appointment is Tuesday at two?" This confirms information without directly questioning their memory.

When Howard started struggling with managing his medications - something he'd done independently for years - his son didn't take over completely. Instead, he suggested they "organize the pill box together" each week during his regular visits. Howard still made the decisions about timing and dosage, consulting his medication list. At the same time, his son quietly double-checked and helped with the physical sorting. This approach allowed Howard to maintain his role as the manager of his own care while ensuring accuracy and safety.

Recognizing When to Step Back

Part of helping without taking over means recognizing when your assistance isn't needed or wanted. Some days will be better than others. Some tasks will remain manageable while others become challenging.

Pay attention to cues that suggest you're overstepping:

- Frustration or resistance to your offers
- Comments like "I can still do this myself."
- Withdrawal from activities you've tried to help with

The communication principles from Chapter 4 guide these interactions - staying calm, using simple language, and following their lead rather than imposing your timeline or methods.

Remember that this stage won't last forever. As we'll explore in Chapter 11, mid-stage changes will require different approaches and more direct intervention. But for now, your role is that of a supportive partner, helping maintain independence while quietly ensuring safety and success.

The best help often feels invisible to the person receiving it.

Building Bridges Through Everyday Conversations

People in early-stage dementia often worry about being treated differently once others know about their diagnosis. Maintaining natural, respectful interactions helps preserve important relationships and supports emotional well-being during a time of significant adjustment.

The fear of social isolation runs deep during this stage. Many people notice their own cognitive changes before others do, leading to anxiety about how friends and family will react. When conversations become strained or people start speaking to them differently, it confirms their worst fears about losing their place in their social world.

Your approach to everyday conversation can either build bridges or create distance.

Keeping Conversations Natural

Continue to include them in group conversations and social activities rather than having side conversations about them or excluding them from decisions. The subtle shift from talking with someone to talking about them in their presence damages dignity and connection.

Allow for natural pauses and repetition without making it obvious or awkward. When someone repeats a story or question, acknowledge it gracefully rather than pointing out the repetition. A simple "That's interesting" or "I can see why that stuck with you" validates their sharing without creating embarrassment.

Focus on their interests and experiences rather than their difficulties. Ask about topics they've always enjoyed discussing - grandchildren, hobbies, past careers, or current events they follow. These conversations draw on preserved knowledge and help them feel valued for who they are, not defined by what they're struggling with.

Grace had been part of a weekly book club for fifteen years. When she began having trouble following complex plot lines and occasionally repeated comments she'd made earlier in the discussion, some members weren't sure how to respond. The group leader made a simple adjustment: she started each meeting with a brief recap of the previous week's discussion. She encouraged everyone to share their favorite passages rather than focusing on detailed analysis. Grace remained an active, valued member of the group, contributing her insights on characters and themes, and the structure naturally supported her participation.

Conversation Strategies That Work

Use the communication principles from Chapter 4 in natural ways. Speak clearly and give people time to process, but don't make it obvious that you're adjusting your style. These techniques should feel like a patient, thoughtful conversation rather than a special accommodation.

Build on their contributions: When someone shares a memory or observation, ask follow-up questions that help them elaborate. "What was your favorite part about that job?" or "How did that make you feel?" shows genuine interest and helps them stay engaged.

Create opportunities for them to help others: People in early stages often have wisdom and experience to share. Ask for their advice about situations you're facing or invite them to help with tasks they're still capable of managing.

Handle confusion with grace: When someone loses track of a conversation or seems confused, gently guide them back without drawing attention to the confusion. "We were talking about your garden - how are the tomatoes doing this year?" redirects naturally.

Managing Group Dynamics

Sometimes the biggest challenge isn't the person with dementia, but helping others in the group adjust their expectations and responses. As we discussed in Chapter 8, managing emotions in group situations requires patience and understanding from everyone involved.

Lead by example: Your calm, inclusive approach shows others how to interact respectfully.

Provide gentle guidance: If someone in the group seems unsure how to respond to repetition or confusion, model appropriate responses or have a brief private conversation about helpful approaches.

Focus on connection over perfection: The goal isn't perfect conversation - it's maintaining meaningful relationships and social connection.

These everyday interactions matter more than you might realize. As we'll explore in the next chapter on mid-stage changes, the nature of communication will evolve. Still, the foundation of respect and genuine interest you build now will support the relationship's continuity throughout the journey.

Connection happens in ordinary moments.

Walking Beside Someone in Transition

Perhaps the most challenging aspect of early-stage support is helping someone navigate the emotional impact of recognizing their own cognitive changes. This awareness can bring grief, fear, and frustration, requiring a patient, compassionate response.

Unlike the behavioral challenges we discussed in Chapter 9 about sundowning, early-stage emotional struggles often center on the person's awareness of what they're losing. They notice when they can't find words as easily, when familiar tasks become confusing, or when they repeat themselves in conversation.

This awareness creates a unique kind of suffering.

Honoring Their Experience

Acknowledging their feelings without trying to fix or minimize them provides the most meaningful support. When someone says, "I feel like I'm losing myself," responding with "You're fine, don't worry about it" dismisses their very real experience. Instead, try "That sounds really difficult" or "I can see how scary that would be."

Providing reassurance about your continued relationship and support addresses one of their deepest fears - that people will abandon them as their abilities change. Simple statements like "I'm not going anywhere" or "You're still the same person I care about" carry tremendous weight during times of uncertainty.

Helping them focus on what they can still do and enjoy balances acknowledgment of loss with recognition of remaining capabilities. This isn't about false cheerfulness, but about helping them see the full picture of their current abilities alongside the changes they're experiencing.

Samuel became increasingly frustrated when he couldn't remember the names of his grandchildren's teachers or mixed up details from recent family events. During one visit, he told his daughter, "I feel like I'm disappearing bit by bit." Rather than reassuring him that everything was fine, she sat with him quietly and said, "That sounds really frightening. I can't imagine how hard this must be." They spent the afternoon looking through photo albums, with Samuel sharing stories from his childhood that he remembered vividly. By the end of the visit, he seemed lighter, saying, "I may not remember everything, but I remember what matters most."

Walking the Emotional Journey Together

The communication strategies from Chapter 4 become especially important during emotional conversations. Speaking calmly, allowing silence, and following their lead helps create space for difficult feelings without overwhelming the interaction.

Sit with uncertainty: You don't need to have answers for their fears about the future. Your presence and willingness to listen often matter more than solutions.

Validate their observations: If they notice they're struggling with something, acknowledge their awareness rather than minimizing it. "You're right, that task has gotten harder," shows respect for their insight.

Share your perspective gently: While you shouldn't dismiss their concerns, you can offer your viewpoint. "I still see so much of who you've always been" or "Your sense of humor hasn't changed at all" provides balance.

Practical Emotional Support

Create opportunities for success: Plan activities that draw on their preserved abilities and interests. Successful experiences help counterbalance frustrations with more difficult tasks.

Maintain normalcy: Continue treating them as the capable adult they are, even as you acknowledge changes. This balance prevents both denial and premature dependency.

Share the load: Let them know they don't have to manage these changes alone. "We'll figure this out together" transforms isolation into partnership.

The emotional aspects of early-stage support often require the same patience and grace we discussed for handling repetition in Chapter 5. People need time to process their changing reality, and they may return to the same fears and questions repeatedly as they work through their feelings.

Remember that supporting someone through this transition isn't about making their difficult feelings disappear - it's about ensuring they don't face those feelings alone.

Your presence matters more than your words.

Mid-Stage Changes - What Surprises Helpers

Care Through Life's Changing Seasons

THE MIDDLE STAGE OF dementia brings changes that can catch helpers off guard, not because they're dramatic, but because they're subtle and gradual. What worked last month might not work this month, and what seems like a small adjustment can make a significant difference in someone's comfort and well-being.

Unlike the early stage we explored in Chapter 10, where maintaining connection felt more straightforward, mid-stage support requires a different kind of flexibility. You'll notice shifts in how your loved one processes information, makes decisions, and handles daily tasks. These changes don't happen overnight, which is why they can surprise even experienced helpers.

Key changes that emerge during mid-stage:

- Physical tasks that were once automatic now require gentle guidance or assistance

· Decision-making becomes more challenging, even for simple choices

· Personal care needs increase, but dignity and independence remain important

· Familiar routines may need adjustments to remain effective

Elizabeth had been helping her neighbor Connor with grocery shopping for months without any issues. He would make his list, they'd walk through the store together, and he'd make his own choices about brands and quantities. But recently, Elizabeth noticed he'd stand frozen in the cereal aisle, overwhelmed by the dozens of options. What surprised her wasn't that he needed help - it was how a simple solution made all the difference. Instead of asking "What cereal do you want?" she started offering two choices: "Would you like your usual cornflakes or something different today?" This small change turned a stressful situation into a manageable one, and Connor felt capable and involved in the decision.

The Art of Simplifying Without Infantilizing

Mid-stage dementia care requires walking a delicate line between providing necessary support and preserving adult dignity. The communication skills from Chapter 4 become even more crucial now, as you'll need to adjust your approach while maintaining respect and warmth.

Breaking down complex tasks into smaller steps helps tremendously. When Connor struggled to get dressed, Elizabeth learned to lay out his clothes in the order he'd put them on, rather than simply pointing to the closet.

She discovered that too many choices created anxiety, but having everything ready in sequence helped him maintain his morning routine with confidence.

Effective mid-stage support strategies:

· Offer limited choices instead of open-ended questions

· Break multi-step tasks into single actions

· Use visual cues alongside verbal instructions

· Allow extra time for processing and response

The repetition and confusion we discussed in Chapter 5 often increases during this stage. Still, your patient responses remain just as important. Elizabeth found herself answering the same questions about dinner plans multiple times each afternoon. Even so, she noticed that her calm, consistent responses helped Connor feel secure rather than frustrated.

Physical Changes and Safety Considerations

Balance and coordination may become concerns during mid-stage dementia. Simple environmental modifications can prevent falls and help maintain independence longer. Elizabeth added a sturdy chair in Connor's bedroom so he could sit while putting on his shoes and socks. She also removed small rugs that could cause tripping.

Safety modifications that preserve independence:

· Install grab bars in bathrooms

· Improve lighting in hallways and stairs

- Remove clutter from walking paths
- Consider medication management systems

Personal care becomes more involved, but the dignity-focused approach from Chapter 6 remains essential. Elizabeth learned to give Connor privacy while staying nearby for assistance. She'd start his shower running and lay out towels, then step out. At the same time, he began washing, checking back periodically to offer help with harder-to-reach areas.

These mid-stage changes prepare us for the deeper presence and connection that becomes central in later-stage care, which we'll explore in our final chapter.

Rewiring Human Connection for Tomorrow

Mid-stage dementia often brings shifts in how someone processes and responds to conversation. They may struggle to find words, lose track of thoughts mid-sentence, or seem to drift away during discussions. These changes don't mean connection is impossible - they mean it's time to adjust your approach.

The communication skills we explored in Chapter 4 become even more essential now, but they need refinement. What worked during early-stage support may feel clumsy or overwhelming as cognitive changes progress. Understanding these shifts helps you maintain meaningful relationships without frustration.

Common mid-stage communication changes:

- Word-finding becomes more difficult, leading to frustration or withdrawal

· Following complex conversations or multiple topics becomes challenging

· Non-verbal communication and emotional connection remain strong

· Attention spans may shorten, but meaningful moments still happen

Lucas used to love discussing current events with his daughter when she visited. Lately, though, he'd become quiet during these conversations, sometimes looking confused or changing the subject entirely. His daughter worried she was boring him or that he no longer enjoyed her visits. Then she realized what was happening: the rapid pace of news topics and complex political discussions was too much to keep up with. When she shifted to talking about one simple topic at a time - his garden, a funny story from work, or memories from her childhood - Lucas became animated again. He couldn't follow the news anymore, but he could absolutely connect with stories and emotions.

The relationship was still there; it just needed a different pathway.

Finding New Conversation Rhythms

The repetition we discussed in Chapter 5 often increases during the mid-stage. Nevertheless, your patience and understanding responses become even more valuable. Instead of viewing repeated questions as problems to solve, consider them as opportunities for connection and reassurance.

Olivia noticed that her husband, Lucas, asked about their son's upcoming visit multiple times each day.

Rather than becoming frustrated, she learned to respond warmly, each time, often adding a small detail: "Yes, David is coming Sunday. He's bringing those cookies you like." This approach turned repetitive questions into moments of anticipation and joy rather than sources of stress.

Effective mid-stage conversation strategies:

- Focus on feelings rather than facts
- Use photos or objects to support discussions
- Allow natural pauses without rushing to fill silence
- Celebrate small moments of clarity and connection

When Words Fail, Connection Continues

As verbal communication becomes more challenging, physical presence and emotional attunement become increasingly important. The gentle touch techniques from Chapter 6 and emotional regulation skills from Chapter 8 prove invaluable during this stage.

Olivia discovered that her father, Lucas, responded beautifully to music, even when conversation became difficult. She'd bring her phone and play songs from his era, watching his face light up as he hummed along or tapped his fingers. These musical moments created a connection that didn't require words but felt deeply meaningful to both of them.

Touch remains a powerful communication tool. A gentle hand on the shoulder, holding hands while sitting together, or offering a warm hug can convey love and support more effectively than words during challenging moments.

Building Toward Deeper Presence

These mid-stage adjustments in communication and connection prepare you for the profound importance of presence that characterizes later-stage care. While cognitive abilities may continue to change, the human need for connection, comfort, and love remains constant.

The skills you're developing now - simplified communication, patience with repetition, and non-verbal connection - will serve you well as you learn to provide meaningful support regardless of cognitive changes. In our final chapter, we'll explore how presence itself becomes the most powerful gift you can offer.

When Guard Rails Matter Most

As dementia progresses, safety awareness diminishes in ways that aren't always obvious. Someone might still seem quite capable in many areas while developing blind spots in others. Recognizing these changes early helps prevent accidents without being overly restrictive.

The fear of "doing it wrong" that we addressed in Chapter 3 often resurfaces when helpers notice these safety changes. You might worry about overstepping boundaries or taking away someone's independence. But creating a safer environment doesn't mean taking control - it means making thoughtful adjustments that preserve dignity while reducing risks.

Common safety changes in mid-stage:

· Judgment about everyday risks becomes less reliable

· Spatial awareness and depth perception may be affected

· Temperature sensitivity and body awareness can change

· Sequencing of familiar tasks may become confused

Sarah seemed perfectly fine managing her daily routine when her son visited on weekends. She could still make tea, tend to her plants, and move around her house confidently. But her son started noticing small things: she'd reach for a hot pan without using a potholder, or she'd step off a curb without looking properly. She wasn't confused or disoriented - she simply wasn't registering these risks the way she used to. Instead of taking over these tasks entirely, her son made subtle environmental adjustments. He moved potholders to more obvious spots, improved lighting near steps, and started gently guiding her arm when they crossed streets. Sarah maintained her independence while staying safer, and she barely noticed the extra support.

Subtle Safety Without Control

The communication principles from Chapter 4 become crucial when addressing safety concerns. Direct warnings like "Be careful!" or "Watch out!" can create anxiety without being helpful. Instead, gentle guidance and environmental modifications work more effectively.

When helping someone navigate potential hazards, prioritize prevention over intervention. Remove throw rugs that could cause trips rather than constantly reminding someone to watch their step. Place frequently used items at easy-to-reach heights rather than repeatedly cautioning about climbing on chairs.

Effective safety strategies:

- Make dangerous items less accessible rather than forbidding their use
- Improve lighting and visibility in key areas
- Create clear pathways free from obstacles
- Use visual cues to highlight important safety information

Temperature and Physical Awareness

Changes in body awareness can catch helpers off guard. Richard noticed that his wife, Sarah, would wear heavy sweaters on warm days or forget to put on a coat in cold weather. Her internal temperature gauge seemed off, but arguing about clothing choices created stress for both of them. Instead, he learned to adjust the home temperature slightly and suggest clothing changes indirectly: "I'm feeling chilly - maybe we should grab sweaters before we go out."

The personal care approaches from Chapter 6 also apply here. When someone's awareness of their physical needs changes, gentle assistance becomes more important. Sarah sometimes forgot to drink water regularly, so Richard started offering her favorite beverages throughout the day rather than reminding her to stay hydrated.

Kitchen and Cooking Considerations

The familiar comforts of cooking that we discussed in Chapter 7 may need safety modifications during mid-stage dementia. Rather than taking over meal preparation entirely, consider gradual adjustments that maintain involvement while reducing risks.

Richard removed sharp knives from easy reach but left safe cutting tools available. He unplugged small appliances after use and moved potentially dangerous items to less accessible cabinets. Sarah could still help with cooking, but within a safer framework.

These safety awareness changes signal the increasing importance of presence and attentiveness, which become central to later-stage care. In our final chapter, we'll explore how your watchful, caring presence becomes the most valuable gift you can offer.

Consistency Beats Flexibility Every Time

In mid-stage dementia, the brain increasingly relies on familiar patterns and predictable sequences. What might seem like rigidity is actually the mind's way of managing complexity. Small disruptions to routine can create disproportionate confusion, while maintaining consistent patterns provides security and confidence.

The routines we discussed in Chapter 7 become even more crucial now, but they require a deeper understanding. This isn't about being inflexible - it's about recognizing that consistency reduces cognitive load and allows someone to use their mental energy for connection and enjoyment rather than constantly figuring out what comes next.

Why routines become essential:

· Daily schedules become anchoring points that reduce anxiety

· Changes in routine can trigger confusion even in familiar environments

· Flexibility should come from helpers adapting to established patterns, not changing them

· Predictable sequences help the brain function more efficiently

Marcus had always been adaptable and easygoing, so his family was surprised when he became distressed if dinner was served at 6:30 instead of 6:00, or if his usual chair was occupied by a visiting grandchild. They initially thought he was becoming difficult or demanding. But his daughter realized this wasn't about control - it was about cognitive load. When everything followed the expected pattern, Marcus could relax and enjoy himself. When things were different, even slightly, his brain had to work harder to make sense of the situation, leaving him tired and anxious. Once the family understood this, they stopped seeing his need for routine as limiting. They began to see it as helpful information. They could still have family gatherings and special occasions; they just made sure Marcus's key routines - his chair, his dinner time, his usual bedtime routine - stayed consistent within those events.

Building on Established Patterns

The communication principles from Chapter 4 apply strongly here. Instead of explaining why routines are changing, focus on maintaining them. Rather than saying "We're eating early today because of the party," simply serve dinner at the usual time and let the party activities happen around that anchor point.

This approach builds on the emotional regulation strategies from Chapter 8. When routines remain consistent, stress levels stay manageable for everyone involved. The sundowning behaviors we explored in Chapter 9 often improve when daily patterns remain predictable.

Flexibility Within Structure

True flexibility in mid-stage care means adapting your approach to work within established patterns rather than changing those patterns. If someone always reads the newspaper after breakfast, continue that routine even if they're no longer actually reading. Sit with them, flip through pages together, or read interesting items aloud. The activity continues to provide comfort and a sense of normalcy.

Strategies for maintaining helpful routines:

- Keep meal times, bedtime, and wake-up times consistent
- Maintain the sequence of morning and evening activities
- Preserve favorite daily activities even if participation changes
- Create predictable transitions between activities

When Flexibility Does Help

The one area where flexibility serves you well is in your response to routine disruptions. When unexpected changes happen - a doctor's appointment, a family emergency, or illness - your calm adaptation helps minimize the impact. Use the soothing communication techniques from Chapter 4 and the emotional support skills from Chapter 8 to navigate these disruptions gently.

Olivia learned that when her father, Marcus, had medical appointments that disrupted his routine, preparing him the night before and maintaining as many familiar elements as possible helped tremendously. She'd bring his usual morning coffee in a travel mug and pack his favorite snacks, creating anchors of normalcy within the disrupted day.

These mid-stage insights about consistency and routine prepare you for understanding how presence itself becomes the most reliable constant in later-stage care, where your steady, caring attendance provides the ultimate anchor point for someone navigating an increasingly confusing world.

Later-Stage Presence - What Still Matters Deeply

When Hearts Speak Without Words

When traditional conversation becomes difficult or impossible, connection doesn't end - it simply changes form. The human need for comfort, recognition, and gentle interaction remains strong even when verbal responses fade. Your presence can provide profound comfort through non-verbal channels that often speak louder than words ever could.

Unlike the mid-stage challenges we explored in Chapter 11, where communication required patience and creativity, later-stage dementia calls for a different kind of presence altogether. The person you're visiting may not remember your name or respond with words, but they can still feel your warmth, kindness, and care.

The Power of Simple Presence

Keira was nervous about visiting her neighbor Edward, whose dementia had progressed significantly since her last visit six months ago. He no longer spoke much and seemed not to recognize most visitors. But when she sat beside him and began humming "Blue Moon" - a song she remembered him singing while working in his garden - his eyes brightened, and he began tapping his fingers on the armrest. They spent the entire afternoon in comfortable silence, with her occasionally humming familiar tunes. Later, his daughter told her it was the most peaceful he'd been all week.

"You didn't need to say a word," she said. "My father felt your kindness."

What Still Connects

Even when cognitive abilities have declined significantly, several pathways to connection remain remarkably intact:

· A gentle, familiar touch can provide immediate comfort and reassurance

· Music from their era or favorite songs can spark recognition and calm

· Simply sitting quietly nearby communicates care and safety

· Soft, soothing voices create a peaceful atmosphere even without conversation

· Familiar scents like favorite perfumes or baking smells can evoke positive feelings

Your Presence Makes a Difference

Research shows that people with advanced dementia can still sense emotional atmospheres and respond to calm, loving energy. When you visit with a peaceful heart and gentle manner, you create an island of tranquility in what might otherwise feel like a confusing world.

Remember the communication principles from Chapter 4: speak slowly, use gentle tones, and maintain eye contact. These remain important even when responses seem minimal.

Practical Ways to Connect

- Hold their hand gently if they seem comfortable with touch
- Share photo albums from their past, describing what you see
- Read favorite poems or Bible verses aloud
- Play music they once enjoyed
- Bring familiar objects that might spark recognition
- Simply sit peacefully together without feeling pressure to fill the silence

When Words Aren't Needed

Edward visited his elderly aunt every Sunday, even though she rarely spoke anymore. Instead of trying to make conversation, he would sit by her window, quietly reading his newspaper while she watched birds outside. Sometimes he'd point out a cardinal or comment softly about the weather. These simple moments created a rhythm of companionship that brought visible peace to both of them.

The beauty of later-stage visits lies in their simplicity.

You don't need to entertain or educate. Your calm presence is a gift.

Trusting Your Heart

Building on everything you've learned about letting go of fear from Chapter 3, trust that your genuine care transcends words and memory. The person may not remember your visit tomorrow, but in the moment, your presence brings comfort and dignity.

Sometimes the most profound connections happen in silence, when hearts recognize hearts and souls touch across the barriers that dementia creates.

Finding Peace Through Gentle Care

In later stages, the goal shifts from stimulation and activity to creating a calm, comfortable atmosphere. This isn't about giving up or doing less - it's about recognizing what truly serves the person now. Your role becomes one of creating a peaceful environment where they can simply be, without pressure to perform or respond.

Unlike the mid-stage approach we discussed in Chapter 11, where maintaining familiar activities remained important, later-stage care requires a gentler philosophy. The person's world has become smaller, and your job is to make that smaller world as peaceful and comfortable as possible.

Creating a Sanctuary of Calm

When Ian came to help with his uncle for the weekend, he initially felt frustrated that all his planned activities - looking through photo albums, playing card games, going for walks - seemed to agitate rather than engage his uncle. Finally, he simply sat with him in the sunny living room, occasionally offering sips of tea and adjusting the cushions behind his back. His uncle dozed peacefully, and when awake, seemed content to watch the birds outside the window.

Ian realized that creating a calm, safe space was exactly the kind of help his uncle needed most.

The Art of Gentle Presence

Your approach should prioritize comfort over stimulation:

- Prioritize their physical comfort with soft lighting, comfortable seating, and gentle temperatures
- Reduce overwhelming stimuli like loud noises, bright lights, or too many people
- Focus on familiar comforts rather than new activities or experiences
- Move slowly and speak softly to avoid startling or overwhelming them
- Allow for plenty of rest without feeling you need to keep them active

Recognizing What Matters Now

Remember the communication techniques from Chapter 4 and the emotional awareness from Chapter 8. These skills remain crucial, but they're applied with an even gentler touch. The person may not engage verbally, but they still respond to kindness, patience, and respect.

Simple Comforts That Make a Difference

The most meaningful help often involves basic comfort measures:

· Ensuring they're warm enough with a soft blanket

· Offering small sips of water or favorite beverages throughout the day

· Playing very soft, familiar music in the background

· Keeping their favorite pillow or stuffed animal nearby

· Maintaining a consistent, quiet routine

When Less Becomes More

Violet discovered this truth when caring for her grandmother. Instead of trying to engage her in conversation or activities, she focused on creating a peaceful afternoon. She dimmed the harsh overhead lights, played gentle classical music, and simply sat nearby doing quiet needlework. Her grandmother, who had been restless all morning, gradually relaxed and spent several hours in peaceful contentment.

Sometimes the greatest gift is simply being present without expectations.

Embracing the Sacred Ordinary

Building on the fear-releasing principles from Chapter 3, accept that later-stage care looks different from what you might have imagined. There's profound beauty in these quiet moments of companionship. You're not failing if conversation doesn't happen or activities don't work.

You're succeeding by creating peace.

Trusting Your Instincts

Your gentle presence communicates what words cannot. When you approach with calm energy and focus on basic comfort, you're providing exactly what's needed. The person may not remember your visit, but in those moments, you're creating an island of tranquility in their world.

The Gift of Peaceful Presence

Later-stage dementia care teaches us that love doesn't require words, activities, or recognition. Sometimes love looks like sitting quietly together, ensuring someone is warm and comfortable, and creating an atmosphere where they can rest peacefully.

This is meaningful help at its most essential.

Navigating Change Together as Families

Later-stage dementia impacts the entire family system, often in ways that aren't immediately visible. Primary caregivers may be exhausted, other family members might be grieving, and everyone is adjusting to profound changes. Your support extends beyond the person with dementia to include understanding and supporting the emotional landscape of everyone involved.

Unlike the mid-stage challenges we explored in Chapter 11, where families were still adjusting to new realities, later-stage care brings deeper complexities. Family members are often processing loss while still providing intensive care, creating emotional burdens that outsiders might not recognize.

Understanding the Family's Journey

Morgan offered to spend Saturday afternoon with her sister-in-law, who had dementia, primarily to give her brother a break. She expected to focus entirely on her sister-in-law's needs, but quickly realized her brother needed just as much support. He felt guilty about leaving, was constantly worried while away, and returned exhausted from trying to pack too much into his few hours of freedom. Morgan learned to text him updates and encouraged him to rest rather than run errands.

Supporting the whole family, she discovered, was just as important as direct care.

The Hidden Emotional Landscape

Family members are navigating complex feelings that may surprise them:

- Acknowledge that family members may be experiencing anticipatory grief as they mourn losses while their loved one is still alive

- Recognize that primary caregivers need both practical help and emotional support to sustain their demanding role

- Understand that family dynamics can become more complex as roles and relationships shift dramatically

Supporting the Primary Caregiver

Building on the emotional awareness skills from Chapter 8, recognize that primary caregivers often carry tremendous emotional weight. They may feel isolated, overwhelmed, or guilty about their own needs and feelings.

When you offer respite care, consider these approaches:

· Send reassuring text messages during your visit: "Everything's going well here."

· Encourage them to truly rest rather than feeling pressure to be productive

· Listen without judgment if they need to express frustration or sadness

· Acknowledge how difficult their daily reality has become

Recognizing Family Grief

Remember the communication principles from Chapter 4 - sometimes the most helpful thing is simply listening. Family members may be grieving the person their loved one used to be, while simultaneously caring for who they are now. This creates a unique kind of ongoing loss that deserves recognition and compassion.

Supporting Extended Family

Children, grandchildren, and siblings often struggle with how to stay connected when visits become difficult. You can help by:

- Sharing positive moments from your visits
- Helping coordinate family visits so multiple people aren't overwhelmed
- Reassuring family members that their presence still matters, even when recognition seems absent
- Offering specific, practical ways they can help

Creating Space for Honest Conversations

Daniel found that his most valuable contribution wasn't just sitting with his neighbor who had dementia, but also providing a safe space for the man's adult daughter to express her fears and frustrations. During their brief conversations when he arrived and left, she could voice concerns she felt she couldn't share with other family members.

Sometimes being helpful means simply listening without trying to fix anything.

The Ripple Effect of Support

When you support the family system, your impact multiplies. A rested primary caregiver provides better care. Reassured family members visit more regularly. Children and grandchildren maintain connections they might otherwise lose.

Your presence creates stability during a time when everything feels uncertain.

Honoring the Whole Journey

Later-stage dementia care isn't just about the person with the diagnosis - it's about honoring the entire family's journey through profound change. Your willingness to see and support everyone affected demonstrates the kind of comprehensive care that truly makes a difference.

This understanding transforms you from a helpful visitor into a vital source of community support.

When Moments Choose Their Witnesses

There is deep meaning in simply bearing witness to someone's experience, especially during vulnerable times. Your presence during later-stage dementia isn't about fixing or improving anything - it's about honoring the person's dignity and ensuring they aren't alone. This kind of presence is a gift both to them and to their family, creating space for whatever each moment brings.

Unlike the more active support we discussed in earlier chapters, later-stage care often calls for a different kind of strength - the strength to simply be present without needing to change or solve anything. This shift from doing to being represents one of the most profound ways you can help.

The Sacred Act of Witnessing

During a particularly difficult evening, Marcus sat with his grandmother, who seemed restless and confused. She kept trying to get up, looking around anxiously, and mumbling that she needed to "go home." He didn't try to redirect or correct her. Instead, he sat nearby, speaking softly and reassuringly: "You're safe. I'm here with you. Everything is okay." Eventually, she settled back in her chair, and they sat together in quiet companionship until she fell asleep.

Later, his mother told him, "She may not remember your visit, but in that moment, she felt safe. That matters more than you know."

Understanding Your Role as Witness

Building on the communication skills from Chapter 4 and the emotional awareness from Chapter 8, your role becomes one of compassionate presence:

· Recognize that your calm presence provides security and dignity during moments of confusion or distress

· Understand that being a witness to someone's experience has inherent value even when you can't change their circumstances.

· Trust that your willingness to be present matters even when you can't see immediate results.

When Nothing Is Everything

Remember the principle from Chapter 3 about letting go of the fear of doing things wrong. In later-stage dementia care, your greatest contribution might be doing very little - but doing that little with tremendous love and patience.

Sometimes the most profound help looks like:

· Sitting quietly while they rest

· Offering gentle reassurance during moments of confusion

· Simply being a calm, steady presence during difficult times

· Maintaining their dignity when they're most vulnerable

The Ripple Effect of Presence

Your willingness to bear witness extends beyond the person with dementia. Family members often find deep comfort knowing their loved one isn't alone during difficult moments. When you're present for the hard times, you're sharing a burden that families carry every day.

Trusting the Moment

Elena discovered this truth while staying overnight with her elderly neighbor. Around midnight, the woman woke up confused and frightened, calling for her mother. Elena didn't try to reorient her or explain that her mother had died decades ago. Instead, she sat on the edge of the bed, held her hand, and spoke gently about feeling safe and loved. Within minutes, the woman relaxed and drifted back to sleep.

The gift wasn't in the explanation - it was in the presence.

Sacred Ordinary Moments

These moments of witness often happen during the most ordinary times: while someone naps in their chair, during quiet afternoons when conversation has faded, or in the peaceful minutes before sleep. Your presence transforms these simple moments into something sacred.

The Honor of Being Chosen

When families trust you to be present during vulnerable times, they're offering you a profound honor. You become part of their loved one's story during a chapter when dignity and companionship matter more than any activity or intervention.

This is meaningful help at its deepest level - being fully present for whatever each moment holds.

When Hearts Speak Without Words

The absence of an obvious response doesn't mean there's no connection. Love, care, and human warmth transcend the limitations that dementia creates. Your gentle presence, kind words, and patient care contribute to their overall sense of well-being, even when they can't express recognition or gratitude. This understanding can sustain you when helping feels one-sided.

Unlike the more reciprocal interactions we explored in earlier chapters, later-stage relationships require a different understanding of connection. The person may not smile back, say thank you, or show obvious signs of enjoying your visit. But connection happens at levels deeper than words or visible responses.

Recognizing Hidden Connection

Charlotte continued visiting her longtime friend even after she stopped recognizing her and rarely spoke to her. During one visit, she was reading aloud from a book they had both enjoyed years earlier when her friend suddenly reached over and patted her hand - the first intentional gesture she had made in months. "I don't think she knew who I was," Charlotte later reflected, "but something in her recognized kindness, recognized care. That connection was real, even if it wasn't the same as before."

These moments remind us that relationships continue even when they look completely different than before.

Understanding Invisible Impact

Building on the communication principles from Chapter 4 and the presence techniques we've discussed throughout this chapter:

· Connection exists beyond verbal acknowledgment or visible recognition through energy, tone, and gentle care

· Your care contributes to their overall sense of safety and comfort in ways that may not be immediately apparent

· The relationship continues to have meaning even when traditional markers of connection have disappeared

When Love Speaks Silently

Remember the emotional awareness skills from Chapter 8. The person with dementia may not be able to process or express emotions in familiar ways. However, they can still sense the emotional atmosphere you create. Your calm, loving presence becomes a gift that operates below the level of conscious recognition.

Trusting the Unseen

Sometimes, connection reveals itself in subtle ways:

- A moment of calm during your visit
- Relaxed breathing when you speak softly
- A brief look that seems to hold recognition
- Physical stillness after periods of restlessness
- Peaceful sleep following your time together

These signs may be fleeting, but they indicate that your presence matters.

The Deeper Gift

Kevin learned this truth while caring for his neighbor with advanced dementia. For months, the man showed no signs of recognizing him or responding to conversation. One afternoon, as Kevin was preparing to leave, the man looked directly at him. He smiled - just for a moment - before returning to his distant gaze. Kevin realized that his regular visits had been creating islands of familiarity and safety, even when no outward response was visible.

Sustaining Your Heart

When you understand that connection transcends obvious responses, you can continue showing up with hope and purpose. Your care isn't wasted when someone doesn't remember your visit or thank you for coming.

Every moment of gentleness matters.

The Eternal Nature of Love

Drawing from the fear-releasing wisdom of Chapter 3, trust that love and care have their own power independent of recognition or response. The person's spirit, their essential humanity, can receive care even when their cognitive abilities cannot process it consciously.

Moving Forward with Confidence

Later-stage dementia doesn't end the possibility for meaningful connection - it transforms it. Your presence matters through gentle touch, familiar music, and simply being there. Focus on comfort rather than engagement, creating peaceful environments over stimulating activities. Remember that you're supporting not just the person with dementia but their entire family system.

Most importantly, trust that connection and love transcend the limitations of dementia, continuing to provide comfort even when responses are minimal or absent.

Conclusion

When you first picked up this book, you may have been feeling that familiar mixture of willingness and worry - wanting to help someone with dementia but fearing you might somehow make things worse. Perhaps you were facing an upcoming visit, a weekend of caregiving, or simply wondering how to support a friend or family member navigating this journey.

This book exists to bridge that gap between caring and confidence. It was written for everyday people who don't need to become experts, but who do need to feel equipped. The vision has always been simple: to remove the fear and guesswork from dementia caregiving so that more people feel empowered to offer the kind of meaningful, short-term support that makes an enormous difference.

Dementia touches millions of families, but the ripple effects extend far beyond those directly affected. When fear keeps willing helpers on the sidelines, everyone loses - the person with dementia misses out on additional connection and support, primary caregivers remain overwhelmed and isolated, and potential helpers carry the weight of wanting to do something but not knowing how.

This book was designed to change that dynamic. Not by turning you into a professional caregiver, but by helping you understand that your natural instincts, combined with some practical guidance, are more than enough for the short-term support situations you're likely to encounter.

The goal was never perfection. It was confidence.

Confidence to sit with someone for an hour without panicking about repetitive questions. Confidence to help with an afternoon without feeling responsible for entertainment or improvement. Confidence to step in for a weekend knowing that maintaining calm consistency matters far more than having all the answers.

What You've Learned

Throughout these pages, several key themes have emerged that reshape how we think about dementia caregiving:

· Dementia is a journey, not a single event. Understanding what dementia looks like day to day helps normalize the experience and reduces the shock of unexpected moments. Repetition, confusion, and changes in routine are part of the landscape, not emergencies requiring immediate solutions.

· Your role as a helper is both smaller and larger than you think. Smaller because you're not responsible for managing dementia or fixing problems. Larger because your calm presence and familiar face provide security and connection that no medical intervention can replace.

· Fear of "doing it wrong" often prevents more help than actual mistakes do. The worry about saying the wrong thing or handling a situation imperfectly keeps many caring people from offering support that would be genuinely valuable. Most "mistakes" are easily recoverable.

· Communication that soothes focuses on tone over content. How you say something matters more than getting the words exactly right. A gentle voice, an unhurried pace, and a willingness to follow the conversation wherever it leads create more comfort than perfect responses.

· Each stage of dementia offers different opportunities for connection. Early stages allow for more complex interactions and shared activities. Later stages call for simpler presence and sensory comfort. All stages benefit from consistent, gentle human connection.

Your Greatest Takeaways

As you close this book and prepare to put these ideas into practice, carry these essential truths with you:

Your willingness to help is already your greatest qualification. No amount of training can substitute for genuine care and the desire to support someone. The fact that you picked up this book and read this far demonstrates that you already possess the most important quality needed for helping: a heart that cares.

Simple routines and familiar comforts provide profound peace. In a world where dementia creates increasing uncertainty, maintaining predictable patterns becomes deeply therapeutic. Your role in preserving these routines provides stability that helps reduce anxiety and confusion.

Love and connection transcend cognitive changes. Even as dementia progresses and communication becomes more challenging, the human need for connection remains intact. Your presence, gentle touch, familiar voice, and patient attention communicate care in ways that go beyond words.

Calm consistency trumps complicated interventions. The most sophisticated care techniques pale in comparison to the power of a steady, unhurried presence. Your ability to remain emotionally regulated when someone else is confused or distressed provides the kind of grounding that helps restore peace to difficult moments.

Your Next Steps

Now comes the important part: taking action. Here's how to move forward with confidence:

Start small with one-hour visits to build confidence. Don't wait until you feel completely ready or until a crisis demands your help. Begin with short, low-pressure visits that let you practice the principles you've learned while gradually building your comfort level.

Focus on creating calm rather than accomplishing tasks. Shift your definition of successful helping from getting things done to maintaining a peaceful atmosphere. If your presence helps someone feel more relaxed, you have made a significant difference.

Remember that showing up matters more than getting everything right. Your presence communicates care in ways that perfect technique cannot. The person you're helping benefits more from your consistent, imperfect attention than they would from sporadic, flawless assistance.

Trust that your care and presence make a real difference. Even when you can't see immediate results or when interactions feel repetitive or confusing, your contribution matters. The security of having a caring person nearby provides benefits that may not be immediately visible, but they are profoundly real.

A Personal Reflection

As I finish writing this book, I find myself thinking about all the conversations I've had with people who wanted to help but felt paralyzed by the possibility of making mistakes. These weren't uncaring people. They were people who cared deeply but felt overwhelmed by uncertainty.

What changed everything was understanding that these challenging moments, while difficult, were manageable. They were part of the human experience, not crises requiring perfect responses.

If this book has helped you move from fear to confidence, from paralysis to action, from worry about perfection to focus on presence, then it has succeeded beyond my hopes.

You now have the foundation to step forward with confidence. You understand that your heart to help, combined with practical guidance and realistic expectations, creates exactly the kind of support that transforms lives - both for those with dementia and for their families.

The person you help may not remember every detail of your time together, but they will carry the feeling of being cared for. The primary caregiver may not be able to express their gratitude adequately. Still, they will feel the relief of knowing they're not alone.

Dementia changes many things, but it doesn't change the fundamental human need for connection, dignity, and care. Your willingness to provide those things - imperfectly, perhaps, but genuinely - makes you part of a network of support that sustains families and communities through one of life's most challenging journeys.

As a special thank you for caring about connection and choosing this guide, a free bonus resource is included below. Simply scan the QR code to access and download your printable companion materials.

The world needs more people like you - people who care enough to learn, who are willing to step in despite uncertainty, who understand that love and presence matter more than expertise.

You are ready. You have always been ready.

The person who needs your help is waiting, and they don't need you to be perfect. They just need you to show up.

Go forward with confidence. You've got this.

A Warm Invitation From The Author

********REVIEW********

DEAR WONDERFUL READER,

Thank you deeply for journeying with me through the pages of this book. Every word was written with you in mind – crafted to inspire, comfort, or simply bring joy into your day.

If this book has touched your heart, made you smile, or gently enriched your life, would you consider sharing your thoughts in a brief review?

Your words hold extraordinary power – not only do they help others find the book, but they also inspire me profoundly as an author, guiding and nurturing my creative path forward.

It would mean the world to me if you took just a moment to leave your honest reflections. Whether a few words or several lines, every review makes an enormous difference.

If you're willing

When you have a moment, you can return to where you found this book and leave a few genuine lines:

What helped you most?

What felt reassuring or practical?

Who would you recommend this book to?

Or, if it's easier, you can use this link:
https://www.amazon.com/review/review-your-purchases/?asin=B0GMDDJSM6

Thank you for caring enough to learn, and for showing up in the lives of others.

Warmly,
Natalie Mills
Author of *Mindful Midlife Reset*

Made in the USA
Monee, IL
04 November 2026

67383860R00105